What Will Not Kill You...

A Memoir

What Will Not Kill You...

A Memoir

By

Annemarie Duparc

Strategic Book Publishing and Rights Co.

Strategic Book Publishing and Rights Co.
12620 FM 1960, Suite A4-507
Houston TX 77065
www.sbpra.com

ISBN: 978-1-62212-807-5

For Philippe, Stephen and Richard, my beloved sons.

à Jacqueline, mon amie
en témoignage de mon
affection.

Renée

My sincere thanks to Sophie, my daughter-in-law and friend, without whose suggestion this memoir would never have been published.

Table of Contents

PART ONE

I was born seventy-nine years ago. I have been told I look twenty years younger. That's because my life started at sixty. Here is why.

My very first memory is of a lavender and purple living room carpet. I must have been two or three years old. I remember the floor being very close to my eyes. Women (a nurse, the maid) were running around carrying basins and telling me to get out of the way. This was a room I was not allowed to enter anyway, but in the panic and confusion, I somehow found myself in there. I could hear my mother retching in another room. I think she was pregnant with my second younger sister. I was gripped by terror and anxiety. Something terrible was happening. Was my mother being hurt? Was she very ill? I don't know if I had a concept of serious illness in those days. Strangely enough, for me this was a traumatizing episode, and surely one of some significance in the life of my mother. It was never referred to by my parents. Mother always made it abundantly clear that pregnancy was a burden.

Before my sisters and I had children of our own, I recall Mother saying that when she carried us she suffered from *vomissements incoercibles*, uncontrollable vomiting, which sounded absolutely horrendous to me. It must have been at that moment I started thinking there were some very negative aspects to motherhood. Perhaps the fact that being with child was due to a sexual intimacy she didn't really relish made pregnancy unpalatable to my mother, so to speak. Grandmother certainly never exhibited any joy with her brood of eleven either. Come to think of it, in those years, amongst the devout Catholic ladies I knew, the attitude was more that maternity was foisted on women and that they better make the best of it. My own mother dwelled on the debilitating aspects, and as far as she was concerned, there were no rewards.

My parents, my three sisters, and I lived in an apartment above my maternal grandparents' place at that time. The whole house had originally been a Victorian mansion. My grandparents had eleven living children left out of sixteen. The other five were deceased before I was born. Of those, the one most often mentioned died of the Spanish flu right after the First World War. He had been a soldier. He was twenty-one. I also know that the youngest of the sixteen not to survive were twins who died in childbirth. Originally, the family had occupied the whole house, which was later divided into a triplex when only one unmarried daughter remained at home. It was a beautiful residence. My most vivid recollection is of the bathroom, which had tiles and fixtures coloured green — not turquoise, not aqua, but a tint reminiscent of stagnant water, which was very unusual and rare in those days and stunning in our small town. Glamorous people in big cities probably had them.

The house also had a conservatory to one side where my grandmother used to sit in winter. It was of grayish marble, and full of sun. In warm weather she would sit on the huge front verandah in a rocking chair and watch the world go by. And most of the population did go by, since the house was on Main Street across from the imposing parish church. My grandparents were well enough to-do: Grandfather owned a higher quality furniture store, and drove huge Chrysler automobiles, which my uncles regularly demolished.

It was unfortunate that we lived above my grandparents, because Grandmother was not fond of my sisters and me. She never wanted to see us, and after bringing sixteen children into the world, it was understandable. I think also that she was ashamed of the way we dressed, for she had very good taste and was very proud. She sewed all of her daughters' clothes, who were known to be the best-dressed girls in town. Mother, on the other hand, did not have the energy for that kind of thing. She did not care what we wore, as long as it was cheap. She accepted hand-me-downs for us with great satisfaction. I think the idea at the time was that Father was a struggling young doctor.

My parents, like all professionals and upper-middle class people of that period, had a maid. Father would spot the young women when he went to deliver babies at farms in the countryside. They were glad to find work in a home in town, those farmers' daughters from huge families where the boys toiled with the land. The maid must have been there to do the cleaning of the house and other chores as well as babysit us. My mother did all the cooking. I don't remember her ever doing anything else. Our laundry was sent out. I would wonder why we didn't have a washing machine like every other household. Those were the days when you had to put the wet clothes through a wringer. An arduous job, I thought, as I sometimes observed our neighbour labour at her wash. I know my grandmother's laundry was done at home. Our maid must have been paid peanuts, but I assume it was even cheaper to send the laundry out. I'm sure at some point I asked my mother why we didn't have a washing machine like everyone else. Her answer must have been, "It's too hard to do. I'm weak, as you know."

That is how my mother perceived herself: devoid of physical strength. Anything to do with the household and family was an effort, although she mentioned that they did go skiing up north in the first years of the marriage.

My parents alternated with the maid for nights out. They stepped-out every second day of the week. There was no television; fortunately, they were both avid readers. I hated those evenings when we were left with the maid. I felt anguished. I felt abandoned. I believe that anxiety stemmed from the sense I had that our parents did not love us. At all times, we children were put to bed very early, to get us out of the way. I knew our friends never went to bed at seven o'clock like us. I use to lie there, frustrated. I would have liked to see my mother all dressed up. She was so beautiful.

In those days, the main meal of the day was at noon, and the men came home to eat it. My grandmother always served soup first before the main dish. I don't think my mother bothered with the soup; that was reserved for the evening meal, which was always lighter fare. In the mornings, she wore, like every other woman, a cotton house-dress for "working," and then around one o'clock she was free for the afternoon. She would change into a smart outfit and go out. I imagine she shopped at the butcher and the grocer every day, although milk and bread were delivered to the house. There were no supermarkets at first, but then one day an A & P was opened on Main Street. That store did not offer that marvel which some years later another company would provide in its grocery stores: an automatic door. Whenever we went for a short stay with my cousins, who lived in the big city, we accompanied my aunt to that supermarket for the sole purpose of standing in front of that door and seeing it open by itself to let us inside.

These cousins, five of them, were far from being well-off. The Depression had done its job on their father, who came from a wealthy family. Their first floor flat was dingy compared to our house, but I envied them. Their playground, the big city, was so much more fun than the country fields where we romped after we moved from my grandparents' house to our own place. As long as we dwelled in the upstairs apartment of their mansion, we were confined for our outdoor games to a piece of lawn at the back, blocked at the bottom by an old, disused barn and on the right by a chain link fence which separated us from the grounds of the Anglican church next door. Against that side of the fence were apple trees.

One day, yielding to my younger devilish siblings' pressing suggestion – I was a very obedient little girl, and leaving our yard was a no-no – I went over the fence and climbed a tree. Just as I was about to pick an apple, I heard a deep, loud voice tell me not to touch the apples and to come down immediately. It was a policeman. I was petrified. I was sure I was going to jail, because he had shouted "Thieves!" He marched us to our house, all along reprimanding us in a very stern voice. I was terrified at what Grandmother's and Father's reactions would be. I knew neither Mother nor Grandfather would care, although I never sensed that anybody thought the whole incident was funny. We were probably grounded and Father probably had to pay a fine. Strange that the Anglican people had called the police; I must have been six at the most. Did they eat their apples? Were they McIntoshes (the only valuable kind in those days)? I had never seen them picking the fruit.

My siblings and I weren't allowed to leave that back enclosure because it was deemed too dangerous for us to play on the street. One side of it was wide open, a paved road which led to the garages attached to my grandparents' dwelling, and then further back to those of the electricity company. At the bottom, opposite the house, was a barn which opened on the opposite side onto a field belonging to a family who raised turkeys. One time I ventured to "the other side" and discovered what appeared to me, at my age, to be creatures twice my size, and because of their odd appearance, like monsters. I started running, seeking to escape. One of them, probably the male, came after me and pecked at me. Fortunately, my fear gave me wings and strength and I was able to avoid a full-fledged attack, but I never forgot the incident.

My two sisters regularly escaped the backyard. There was absolutely nothing for us to do there except play with our dolls. There was no apparatus like a swing or a trapeze, just grass. Being a good little girl, I never went with them. I was bored out of my mind, with that usual sad, empty feeling.

After our youngest sister was born, our parents started renting a cottage for the summer but they somehow always rented one where there were no children our age. I did not like playing with my siblings. I did not love them. Affection is not something that flourished in our family. I believe, and it certainly conformed to the atmosphere of rejection which was ambient in our home, that Father was very happy to have us all out of the way so that he could bum around in peace, and that Mother was thrilled to have one less human being, and a very hateful one at that, to deal with on a daily basis. True, she had the four of us girls underfoot, but when we were younger there was always the maid. My sisters were always getting in trouble, and I guess I figured if I was obedient, my parents would love me. I did have a reputation for being well-behaved, but it did not do the trick as far as being cherished was concerned. Being in the country, Mother figured we couldn't get into trouble outside the house.

I never really learnt to swim, not well enough to save my life, despite all those summers near a lake. I don't like getting wet, not unless it's a scorcher, but I like going into the ocean where I know there's clean sand under my feet. With fresh water, you never know. Our parents could not swim and never went in the water themselves. They owned bathing suits, but my mother always had some excuse not to join us. When father did wade in, about once a summer, it was quite an event.

Nevertheless, my siblings and I, and the dog, which would go insane when he heard Father's car in the driveway, were very happy when he showed up on a Wednesday afternoon and for a couple of days on the weekends inebriated to various degrees; in our case because he was always full of stories. He was a good *raconteur* with a sardonic touch. The animal was happy because he knew that soon he would go for a ride, perched on the forward end of the boat, ecstatic to share private moments with his master, at first slicing the air with his nose, letting it wash over his panting body, and then lying down, waiting peacefully for hours while the man of the house fished, mostly without any success. It was a rare treat when Father brought back a fish. I could never understand how such impatient an individual could stand still for such a long time in a boat hoping for a catch, often in the heat of a mid-summer afternoon.

We never had company like other people. I guess my mother was always too tired to organize entertaining. To say she was not a partying type is a great understatement. She did not drink or smoke. Her relatives would never have dropped in. Coming to our house simply wasn't a pleasant experience. Father, after a few drinks with the in-laws, would invariably start picking on them, looking for a fight. They were all businessmen on Mother's, side except for the one dentist who had been in the army. Father, in his alcohol-fueled aggressiveness, would always end up bellowing that they were nothing but horse traders.

Once, after having been specifically invited and having reluctantly accepted so as not to hurt Mother's feelings, the relatives arrived to find Father, who had not bothered to dress, greeting them in his long johns. The underwear were opened at the front and back, and he was slobbering drunk, incoherent — dishonor personified. Everyone was embarrassed, and I was mortified to tears. I had so been looking forward to that occasion, if only just to show the neighbours that we too had visitors. That scene is seared forever in my mind. I realized then that it was better if we kept to ourselves.

At the time the fourth sister was born — it must have been because Mother had given birth, nobody ever told us anything – my two other siblings and I were taken away from our home and put into an institution called the Patronage, which was a welfare establishment run by nuns for youths in trouble, I think. The whole place reeked of destitution. Everyone there seemed to resent us. I remember being terrified to the point of diarrhea of being left in what to me felt like my idea of a jail. We had been plucked out of our environment without any explanation. One day, for lunch, we were served our meal on newspapers instead of plates. Outraged, I told my sisters we were not eating on pieces of paper and that we were leaving the premises forthwith. We walked back home, a destination far away and not easy to find for little girls. We must have been crying very hard when we were asked to explain our behaviour, because our parents did not send us back as I feared. It is one of the few times our feelings were ever considered.

There were now four of us, and my parents rented a house in a more residential part of town. We were on a corner, and across the little street running on the side of the house was a magnificent park with two ponds, trees, huge flat rocks, and a bandstand. At the time, it looked immense to me. We were thrilled to have such a vast space to romp in. At the top of the little street was an equally big treed field which held two cows we used to track down. It was like a big adventure, because the place appeared to us like a forest where you could hide and devise all kinds of games.

Across the street from the field was a white mansion which everyone called the White Castle, with real woods behind and where we seldom ventured. Come to think of it, that part of town was full of stately houses.

Across the bigger street which ran along the front of our place, was one of those large homes. It had been divided into a triplex and sat on a small elevation. In the warm weather, the path leading to the two front dwellings was lined with gladiolas on each side. That was a beautiful sight. That street was shaded by very tall old elms and maple trees. It was the right place to live. We could run on the sidewalks and ride our bikes during the summer holidays. One of the dwellings was the home of a family with three children our age, two boys and a girl. The father, whose career as a professional had been foiled by the Depression, was a traveling salesman for a foundry which made kitchen stoves. As such he was seldom home – his son told me recently that he probably had a mistress not far away. The mother was a very accommodating and welcoming woman. It was our second home; in fact, I preferred it to our own household, where I certainly never felt wanted. They loved our new baby sister. They were kind to us, and generous with treats, although they did not have much money. The children did not go to private school as we did, but they were our best friends.

I was secretly in love with the boy who was my age, as later in my teens I was crazy for a gorgeous youth who did not even know I existed. He himself was mooning for the girl, an only child, whose parents were the owners of the triplex, and who lived in the other portion of the big house. She was three years older than me and very good looking.

Further down the street toward downtown was the mayor's relatives' domain. It was a place like those owned by movie stars: there was a tennis court, a pool, huge grounds looked after by a gardener, and all of it was surrounded by a tall wrought-iron fence with stone pillars and a gate like you see in films. The little girl who lived there wore red shoes, unseen in our neck of the woods, and she was a perpetual source of envy for me. I was in awe of it all. Millionaires in our midst! That we were allowed to visit, albeit very seldom inside the mansion, was like a miracle to me. But then, the mayor's sister's husband, the little girl's father, who did not seem to live there, did not have much of a job. He was a cousin of Father's, and my father knew all of their dirty family secrets. I'm sure we looked like ragamuffins to them, but in our teens our friends played tennis with the youths who lived there. One was particularly handsome, but he never noticed me.

I tried my hand at tennis, there and at the convent during the school year, but I was never any good at it because I was too tense and unsure of myself. My very best girl friend in school played tennis until she was in her seventies. That's how she met her husband, and then after their divorce, her successive boyfriends, all belonging to the same club. I would have loved to be reasonably good at it because not having any brothers, that's a dandy way to meet men, as is playing golf. Being so self-conscious, however, I was rather a failure at that as well as skiing and skating. I had a lack of coordination and confidence. Being always uptight, you get tired very quickly.

An Education

Altogether I attended three different boarding schools, all at convents. It was four in total, if you count college in the States, which was also a Catholic institution where I stayed for a year. I can't remember anything about the authorities there. I don't think I boarded in the school where I learned to read and write. It was located on the same street where we lived, just past the park, and it was called the Sisters of the Immaculate Conception. You were taught only cursive writing there, as printing did not exist for humans in those days, at least in my province. My hand was never steady and I've always been ashamed of my handwriting. Later on, of course, I had to teach myself to print. It was very laborious, and the writing was all jiggly. I know some practically illiterate people who have beautiful handwriting. I'm not referring to younger generations who can't read or count, although they can print.

I remember crying in anguish and frustration thinking I would never master learning because reading, arithmetic, and the catechism required such an effort. We had to memorize everything, and at age four, I wasn't used to it. It was work. I had never exercised my mind before, but after a few months I got the hang of it. There was no playful context surrounding the teaching and our mistresses were very strict and stern. Their methodology was infallible, however. You always recognize those who have been schooled in the bosom of religious orders. They have been educated for life.

The second convent we were sent to was ruled by the Sisters of the Presentation. It was located in the lower-town not far from where the Patronage was. It offered classes for day-students as well as boarders. The students who boarded were more or less segregated from the section attended by the pupils who lived at home, who attended something more like a public school. It was a large building where we slept in dormitories, ate in refectories, and played indoors in a big room. There were long hallways and endless staircases, a beautiful chapel, and a reception hall for formal ceremonies, which resembled a ballroom. Outside, there were two yards, one for the little ones and one for the older girls, which today reminds me of a prison yard surrounded by walls on all sides. There were swings, but that was all. The younger students' yard was closed on one side by a chain link fence from which you could see tennis courts where boys played. We would stare at them for long moments, dreaming of freedom.

The rule was that each boarder had the right to a bath — there were no showers — and a hair wash once a month. On that occasion, our heads were ritually combed for lice by the nuns. It hurt. I think I was found to be infested a couple of times. I can still remember spying huge bugs running around on my scalp. Itchy. They were always gotten rid of. Although we didn't know any better, religious boarding schools outside the big city were not what you'd call high-class establishments, but we were taught well. Some of the sisters must have been there for the love of God and therefore possessed of kindness, but I never saw any evidence of it. Sinners, that's what their charges were, except for the *saintes-nitouches, lèche-culs* (brown-noses). My most vivid recollection of my stay in that convent is that of an angry nun grabbing me by the neck and lifting me off the ground. I must have choked, otherwise I would have forgotten the incident, but at the time it did not strike me as unusual treatment. Today I know *sadistic* is the word for it.

Another episode that stands out is one in which Mother's diamond ring disappeared. That was a big deal. We, the offspring, were suspected. Fear. I don't know why, but it occurred to me that maybe my second younger sibling was the one who had purloined it. I searched her clothes and indeed, it was at the bottom of the little purse we wore at the waist under our black serge uniforms. Thief. Shame.

Severe universal reprobation. I don't know what else was done to her, but she had been ostracized all along anyway. In her constant befuddled state, her bloomers were always hanging below her skirt, and she often peed her pants, a source of great embarrassment to her siblings, anger for our parents, annoyance to our keepers, and mockery from our fellow students. No doubt taking the ring was for her an act of revenge on the world, and her way of dealing with our miserable fate. It was certainly a cry for help, as it would be understood today.

This second sister of mine had quite a temper, and did not readily submit to the various injustices which pervaded our family life. One Christmas, when I was perhaps six-years-old and she four, I had the surprise to receive as a present the most beautiful, life-like porcelain doll I had longed for in my dreams, never, but never expecting my wish to come true. It was a miracle. I was overwhelmed with joy, gratitude, and awe. For five minutes. In a rage, this sister grabbed the doll from my hands and smashed it to bits on the floor. She had received as a present the pair of skates which no longer fit me. This incident a perfect witness to Mother's thrift and lack of sensitivity. I remember Father dangling my guilty sibling out of a window in his ire and everyone imploring him not to hurt her. The doll was never replaced.

Mother had a neurotic fear of spending money. Once, we were invited to a little cousin's birthday party and she brought as the sole present old, used, woolen red mitts which had been worn by each of us sisters in turn, and had become stiff and felted from handling snow. I'll never forget the look on my aunts' faces, especially that of the child's mother, who I knew was deeply insulted.

I was not very old, but I could feel her bewilderment. I was deeply ashamed. How could Mother so brazenly expose her cheapness outside our home?

The third school we were sent to, for a short while (I know not for what reason), was located in the village where the snowmobile was invented. Father knew the man, and we had ridden in the prototype, which looked like a tank. I have no idea what religious order we were dealing with this time. Two cousins who lived in a small town nearby were boarding there as well at the time. My memories from that time include the usual black uniform – the style differed from one institution to the other – and a hat for outings to the church. Our parents balked with displeasure at having to pay for an additional item. In that convent, when we took a bath, it was in cold water, and we had to cover ourselves with a cotton tunic so that we wouldn't see our own bodies. As the material got wet and clung to my skin I would start shivering. Torture. To save our souls. My recollection is that we stayed there only a few months.

The next year, it was to still another convent in a small town about fifteen miles from our hometown, where my mother and a couple of other aunts had gone when they were our age. It was an ancient manor built by a railroad tycoon and named after him, up on a hill overlooking the town with a pond on a lower level where swans swam until they all died. Below that, fittingly, were railroad tracks. In the winter we used to ski down that little hill. The nuns made us wear skirts over our ski pants. It was more modest. I thought we looked ridiculous, but it was great fun.

At the beginning I was amongst the juniors. We had our own quarters. I believe we joined the senior girls in grade six. We had a common room arrayed with small lockers which did not lock, in which we could keep small personal effects, like candies. I often stole my cousin's chocolate bars because I was always famished. She knew it was me and despised me for it, but she couldn't prove it, which made her even angrier. I was slightly ashamed, but I was so hungry the temptation was too great. We were never friends. At her age she had no inkling of the startling impoverished circumstances we lived in. After all, wasn't our father a doctor?

It was during the Second World War when food was rationed. The sisters kept our coupons for themselves and ate very well. Our meals were garbage, except for breakfast, which was hot buns and peanut butter, plus coffee made with chicory. That sustained me for the rest of the day because I could not bring myself to ingest what passed for nourishment at the other meals. I was very skinny and at night I used to dream of ham sandwiches. I could not understand the students who stuffed their faces with that slop. They ate better in prisons even in those days, I'm sure. I was so thin that fifty years later at a school reunion, one of my fellow students lifted the jacket I was wearing to see if I had put some meat on those bones. Having always been plump, even during those lean years, she remembered that peculiarity of mine, not eating. I had forgotten it, because now I was struggling against too much weight. That was a direct result of being deprived: as soon as I could afford it, I ate a lot. For years, I was always ready to eat, but now the medication for the tremors has taken care of that. Still, consuming good food is my greatest pleasure.

The other boarders' parents visited quite regularly and brought goodies. They also sometimes took their children to restaurants, or away for certain occasions — I do not remember ever going to an eatery with mine until I was middle-aged. My folks very rarely came to see us and let us come home only when they had to, for Christmas and Easter holydays, and summer vacations. There were a couple of other girls in the same predicament. One of them became my best friend for life although she was in the Anglo program. When some years ago one of her daughters, a godchild of mine, asked me how we had become friends, since we were so different and seemed to have nothing in common, my reply was, "Oh, yes, we both had alcoholic fathers and no one ever came to visit us in the convent."

To be fair, most women didn't drive, and even less owned cars, in those days. It would never have occurred to my mother to take a bus for the purpose of seeing her children. In a way, I was glad my parents did not visit because whenever they showed up, maybe five times in all the years we were there, Father was always drunk and invariably made a scene, which mortified me. One Sunday (it must have been one of those obligatory occasions when we were sent home, Easter perhaps), he was dragged to the parish church for Mass on that special religious day by Mother — I don't know how she succeeded — but that enraged him. I knew it was a bad idea. While the priest was giving his weekly sermon in the pulpit, Father stood up and started shouting abuse at him, *at the priest*, in front of the whole congregation! I wanted to die. Why would my mother risk such a horrifying happening? Father was a mean drunk, and she knew that. When the violence manifested itself in public, we all were witness to what she had to put up with. No doubt every one present felt sorry for her. Little did she think that her children would be marked for life by these debasing, undignified events.

Privately, there were the moments when Father, who hung around in bars 'til the small hours of the morning, would finally come home. Before going to bed, Mother would have phoned the various establishments in town to (as it appeared to me at the time) demand he come home. I now realize she was really just trying to locate him. He ran around. Mother, considering the stress of not knowing where her husband was in the middle of the night, even though he was a doctor, was, strangely enough, always a good sleeper. However, when he finally returned, she could not help but hear him noisily come into their bedroom — the boozy smell alone was enough to wake anyone — and she would invariably tell him to be quiet, that the children were asleep. I am sure she was fully aware what those words would trigger: an explosion of raging fury. *Leave it alone*, I would silently pray, *please*. It was like pouring oil on fire. Beside himself, he would then run around in all the bedrooms, violently tugging at the shades, which would roll up with a racket, punctuated by his loudly cursing what a bloody nuisance we were. We cowered under the blankets, hardly breathing, so as not to attract his attention. In a recent conversation with a cousin, the topic being opera, she mentioned how Father used to play music at top volume on the Gramophone in the middle of the night. She added that her sister, having witnessed his fits of temper, was terrified of him, but luckily he never touched her. Listening to those remarks, I remained silent. The outside world simply had no idea what it was like living under those conditions on a regular basis.

Although I perceived Father as a monster, I could not understand why Mother made things worse by nagging him. It had never worked. Now I know that unconsciously she was signaling what a victim she was. Consequently, as a child I was on constant alert the moment I closed my eyes. All my senses became very acute day and night: for the smell, the look in his eyes, the walk. My powers of observation became such that I could tell in a second his degree of intoxication and its significance for us. That has never left me. I notice my senses are better developed than ninety-nine percent of the population. One day a bunch of us piled into my brother-in-law's car, and right away I smelled something burning. I mentioned it, but no one else noticed the smell. I insisted, and they said I imagined things. When we got out of the car I pointed to smoke that was coming from one of the tires. No one had noticed that either. I reinforced the hostility of a daughter-in-law by hearing her baby waking upstairs in her crib before she did.

Considering his feelings for the clergy, Father was not one to slip money to the nuns for their "good works" either, as other parents did. Consequently, in retribution, we were regularly picked on by our keepers. Actually, my sisters and I looked upon them as jailers. We hated the nuns who, rightly so, found us defiant and hostile. They couldn't stand that we weren't pliable like most of the others, who certainly did not have our reasons to know that everything is not love, faith, and charity. We had never experienced any of those tenets in our personal lives. My objectionable attitude precluded me from being chosen for a membership in the pious society of the *Enfants de Marie*, the Children of Mary. My cousin, though, was president. She was constantly held up to me as a model. Very irritating. I had absolutely no aspirations at being fancied by the nuns in that respect.

My cousin and I were in the same grade, and both achieved the highest marks in class. We were rivals that way. She won in the end. In our graduating year, she came first by half a decimal – in those days we were graded by numbers, not by letters. She had memorized to the last word every single subject which required it. I had given up being that thorough; it was too boring. On graduating day, she was still sixteen and I had become seventeen ten days earlier. Her birthday is on June 25, just after school ended, which meant she finished school when she was younger than me. Somehow, for years that remained very important to me. I was envious. It was one more thing she had that I didn't.

All those years together in the convent, the parents of my cousins (there were two of them, the younger one less of a saint) would be fussed over by the sister who was mistress of discipline, Sister Angealbert, an old, shriveled up nun. The sister especially doted on my aunt, who was always dressed to kill, like a movie star, very elegant, with big hats with floppy rims. She herself had been a student under that nun, who just despised my sisters and me. The despising part I could understand, but why was she so enamoured of my aunt? I finally asked my mother. Years after leaving the convent, it still bothered me. I was sure my cousin, this aunt's daughter, who had married a doctor, had done so much better than me in life. As it turned out, I now triumph and hold my revenge, but in those days my future looked bleak. If mother attended the same convent as our aunt, in the same years, why did Angealbert not recognize the fact and favor us as she did the cousins? "Oh, but I was only there six months," was my mother's answer. Why? "Because I was always fainting. The nuns got tired of it and sent me home."

I guess the first time Mother fainted she received a lot of attention. For a child from a family of eleven, and boarding amongst many others, what a wonderful opportunity to attract attention, to make yourself important. The rest is history. That strategy governed my mother's existence from then on. Resting in bed was her favorite occupation, because, as she claimed, she lacked energy. That was not at all compatible with Father, who was hyperactive and strong as an ox. Of course, then, being physically weak was a woman's prerogative. But many times in his drunken rants Father accused her of being a cold fish in the matter of his conjugal rights. Whenever I heard that, I swore I would never get married. Too much discord. Later on, when I did get married in order to get a roof over my head and by being horny, I remembered my mother's lack of enthusiasm. I abandoned myself to the pleasures of the flesh on demand, and it seemed to be a good solution for harmony in marriage. I was determined, but it didn't last forever. In the meantime I found myself.

The school curriculum was nothing like it is today. I studied Latin for four years, and loved it. Algebra and mathematics in general were a nightmare. I have no memory for numbers, and anything having to do with figures makes my eyes glaze over. I can't believe I gave birth to a son who was practically a mathematical genius. There was no such thing as calculus for us in those days. We had a course in *bienséance*, the rules of etiquette. We were really not groomed to earn a living beyond teaching (not in university), secretariat, nursing, or lab techniques, but another field had just opened to women: social work. However, training for those careers was only accessible if you lived in a big city, unless your parents were willing to pay for your expenses as a college or university student.

I had said I wanted to be a doctor since childhood. I came from a medical family: my paternal grandfather and all the uncles on that side, as well as male cousins, were involved in the profession. My parents never heard my ambition, or if they did, they must have thought it foolish. When my last year of secondary school arrived, they made it very clear that no money would be spent on studies beyond one year. I was to learn English and take a commercial course, not a business course, so that I could earn a living typing and doing shorthand. I was righteously assured that had I been a boy, it would of course have been different, but as I was destined to be married, they weren't about to waste the money on advanced education for someone who could be supported by a husband. Where they thought this husband would come from, I don't know. My sisters and I had no brothers who would bring home school friends to facilitate the meeting of future mates. In fact, my siblings and I didn't have a clue about what made boys tick. I never saw my parents put an ounce of effort into arranging for their daughters to find suitable suitors. The current customs dictated that women had to wait to be asked out by a man. Making phone calls to one of the opposite sex was an exceedingly forward gesture, and it simply was not done. I am still affected by that rule to this day. In those discussions with my parents about my future, what popped in my head was *But what if I never meet someone? Am I condemned to live with you in this hellishly discordant atmosphere which tears me apart?*

Everyone knew I loved studying. The nuns themselves assumed and stated I was meant to go further. I had the reputation of being smart. The realization that my dream of becoming a doctor was not to materialize shattered me. I begged, I cried, I talked about it for weeks. Nothing doing. My mother was the most adamant. She never had any ambition for us, no pride in the fact that I was academically gifted. Why should I do any better than she did? Girls were only meant to get married, have babies, and keep house. Education was wasted money on them. My sisters showed no such scholarly tendencies and had never expressed any preferences. Nevertheless, it was sanctimoniously explained to me that it wouldn't be fair to them if I were allowed to achieve an advanced education because they did not have the means to send all of us to university. Like my female siblings, since I was not a male, I would do a secretarial course and earn a living in an office until I found a husband. Father, being a doctor, meant that applying for financial help was futile, and I wasn't even aware, there being no college in our town, that you could get summer jobs. I had never heard of anyone who did that. In fact, none of my fellow students actually went to university toward a career in the liberal professions. You had to have taken what was known as a "classical course" to achieve that in a private institution, or the nearest seminary if you weren't from the big city. Exceptions were made for young men who went into engineering; they didn't have to study Latin, Greek, or philosophy, as long as they were good at math. Our childhood friend who married one of us made it, although he only had secondary public schooling.

The one other sister who expressed a desire to pursue something other than working in an office wanted to go to art school, which was in the big city. Fortunately for her, she had a godmother who was a millionaire (during the late 1950s). At first, this godmother, when she heard her request, could not believe that she was being asked to subsidize my sister's education. Like everyone else, she assumed that Father, being a doctor, would agree to whatever his children chose for their futures. To be fair, she could not have imagined the lack of concern our parents had for our well-being. After much begging and shedding of tears, and after being explained that borrowing money from the government was out of the question (because if you mentioned on student loan forms that your father was a doctor, you simply did not qualify), my sister's godmother consented to contribute some funds to her studies.

By the time this younger sister had finished secondary school and had a couple of years under her belt at art school, she had learned the ropes, and the possibility of summertime working toward her studies had become familiar to her. She went away to toil in tobacco fields and in big, touristy hotels. Their daughter's determination, and asking for financial help from someone who was not even a relative, thus exposing their callousness, annoyed my parents very much. They did not like the idea that one of their offspring would demean herself by slaving at such lowly labor, mixing with all kinds of people. Father would fly into a rage every time she came home because she was provocative about her lifestyle. She dressed in the *beat* clothes of the day, bringing a whole new world into our midst. My parents did not believe that being an artist was a respectable and legitimate career.

Perhaps as a result of not getting the proper nutrition during the yearly ten months that we spent in boarding school, I used to get these colds which would last for weeks, with fits of bronchial coughing and searing pain in my chest. I did not talk about it, and the authorities were oblivious. When I was much younger, I had frequent bouts of high fever, but that passed. I don't remember the last time I had a high temperature. The regimen at the convent consisted of being awakened by the bell at 5:45 a.m., then ablutions, then making the bed just so, then getting dressed in our uniforms, and then on to chapel for daily Mass. We each brought our missal, which contained the ritual and the various Gospels. I read it like a story all through the ceremony instead of taking part in what the priest was doing at the altar (so boring). I got to know the Gospels by heart. On special days, the choir sang Gregorian chants and cantatas. I was in the choir and enjoyed it very much. I started as a soprano and ended up a contralto, which I prefer. I have lost my voice since I started taking anti-depressants. On the phone I sound much older than I look because of the quiver. Perhaps it's the *essential tremors* that cause it. Very annoying. I still enjoy a very good ear, which is tremendously helpful when speaking different languages.

In boarding school, some fellow students could resort to the "not feeling well today" excuse and be allowed to skip Mass and stay in bed for an additional hour. As it happens, it was the *nouveaux riches,* the pampered ones, who usually took advantage and were granted the privilege. We all knew there was nothing wrong with them. I tried it once, feeling terribly guilty for lying, and was grudgingly given permission: "If you are really sick." To me, sick was having a named disease. Otherwise, it was indulging yourself. Nobody had ever worried about my state of health. That must be the reason I can endure physical pain to a heroic degree with no hysterics and no complaints. Ah, but the anguish that was always eating at me...

I bit my nails into my teens, when pride in my appearance took over. In one of the earlier schools they had covered the end of my fingers with a rag to prevent it. In another one, they had applied something like bitter mustard. It reminds me of my second younger sister who, being left-handed, had her left arm tied behind her back so she would learn to use her right hand to write. It failed.

The happiest time I remember about the years in that particular convent was that come spring, come the month of May, we would attend the early evening religious service dedicated to Mary, mother of Jesus, at the local church. In order to do this, every weekday after our supper, we would walk down to the village, leave the confines of the convent, in ranks of two, supervised by a nun. The weather was soft and warm, the lilacs were in bloom, the air was perfumed, and there were always a bunch of boys hanging out on the porch of the poolroom facing the church. They would emit wolf whistles in our direction the moment they spotted us, to the consternation of our guardian and to our great, half-suppressed exhilaration. We were hustled into the church, but it certainly made our day, although we knew it would feed the "talks" the sisters would regularly have with us regarding the dangers of the outside world.

The locker room for the bigger girls was separated from the sisters' lounge by a thin wall, and we suspected one of them, Sister Alberta, a bully, of leaning on their side of the wall to listen in on our conversations, which consisted mostly of making fun of the nuns or of each other, since we had little contact with the outside world. We did have use of a radio in the common room during free periods, purportedly to hear the latest news about the war, but listening to jazz was forbidden. Music so uninhibited, so prone to improvisation, had to be conducive to moral looseness, years before the sexual revolution and the advent of rock. The reprobates amongst us, of which I was one of the worst, did manage to tune in — we monopolized that corner of the room — to popular music stations whenever there was no supervisor nearby. We were actually obsessed with popular music, with swing, since it meant breaking the rules, and it was our favorite topic of conversation. Sister Alberta would allude to some of the things that were said in the locker room when she picked on me about something or other which had displeased her – it was my attitude really that riled her. When she did so, I would look at her straight in the eye, which enraged her further: "Lower your eyes when I'm talking to you! Have you no shame! *Mauvais esprit!* (disruptive, subversive creature!)." The upbraiding was always done in public, for the purpose of humiliation, which greatly rejoiced my fellow students. Sometimes it did shatter my dignity, sear me to the core, as when it reinforced the reality that my siblings and I were viewed as pariahs due to our wretched family's very public dysfunctional dynamics.

Apparently, the nuns were very concerned about lesbian relationships in our midst. They discouraged close friendships between students, which puzzled me no end, because I had no idea then such a thing existed. I would ask the others why the sisters objected to two girls spending their free time walking together, but I never got a satisfactory answer. I just figured it was another way our guardians had devised to persecute us. There was one girl who would join another girl in bed in my dormitory after lights were out. It would annoy me no end because their whispering kept me awake, but I never noticed they were doing anything else than chatting. Whenever they heard the sister who slept with us in that dorm come in, this student would sneak back to her own bed. I don't think they were ever caught. We were isolated in our little cells by white curtains which formed an enclosure for some privacy. When I found out about Sapphic love a few years later, I wondered if those two had been practitioners.

Finally came graduation day. Even my parents attended, since afterward we had to be brought to our respective homes with our belongings packed in trunks. The other girls were just brimming with joy: no more nuns to talk about the dangers of going out with boys, freedom at last. I was far from being elated. For one thing, there were no males my age where I lived. Our friends across the street had moved to the big city so the boys could attend institutions of higher learning. I did have some sort of a boyfriend from my hometown during that last year who wrote me love poems, which I triumphantly showed to the girls in my class. I was so proud of this literary attention and they were so impressed, given that we had been studying the French symbolist poets Beaudelaire, Verlaine, and Rimbaud. I believe this suitor of mine attended the same seminary as the twins who, come May, served as altar-boys at our daily Mass, to our great titillation. They were our age, brothers to one of the students, and reputedly very talented in the arts, at which they became successful in later life. My boyfriend's precious lyrical letters were surreptitiously passed on to me by a day-girl, a sister of the twin altar-boys. My own paramour was quite good-looking, from the wrong side of the tracks in my hometown, and somehow known to our friends across the street. Wild guy. I can't remember how I met him, but I soon found out that he was two-timing me with our go-between, who being a day-girl, was more accessible. Thus ended our relationship. I never really went out with him except during the one Easter holyday of that last year in the convent. He died very young, remembered by the guys with amusement for being quite dissolute and a bull-shitter. This first romantic betrayal probably contributed greatly to my despair on graduation day. I would totally have forgotten about that relationship were it not for the fact that our childhood friends, when reminiscing about our young adulthood, always mention his escapades somehow derisively, and I experience a kind of relief at not having been too closely associated with him.

My feelings of hopelessness on that last day were akin to post-partum depression. I was facing a void after completing a phase of my existence. Our convent, being in another town, and our having spent summer vacations at cottages in various locations, I had no friends anywhere near our home. My best pal in the convent lived in a city quite far from mine, as did all the cousins my age, and none of us youngsters had the use of cars to travel that far. I was leaving an environment where I had known a certain emotional security, was surrounded by people my age, where confinement assured stability, and where my acknowledged braininess and good marks had given me a certain importance. Now I was being confronted with a vision of endless loneliness, which had somewhat haunted me in recent weeks, although the anticipation of learning how I ranked in the final grading, the graduation ceremony preparations, and general giddiness had kept this apprehension at bay. I was gripped with the terror of it. After receiving my diploma during the ceremony, I started sobbing uncontrollably. I could not stop, shocking everyone around. Father, as surprised as I was by the intensity of my crying, patted me on the shoulders — one of the initial stages of his usual state of inebriation being maudlin sentimentality. It must have appeared to them all that I was overcome by emotion, gratitude towards the nuns, convinced by the speeches, and contemplating a wonderful new life. What I was in fact imagining was that I was a nobody. I was envisaging a grim future, based on the past I had known. I have a very vague recollection of some sort of celebration after the graduation ceremony, obviously at somebody's house (it must have been a day-student's), where boys were present. We had changed into party clothes and to my immense surprise, the males found me attractive and gathered around me, as they would at every social event I attended until my marriage ended.

Since I was destined for secretarial work, my parents wisely figured that I should be more fluent in English. The nuns, who only spoke French, had taught us English as a subject, and I was very good at English grammar and spelling, but conversation in that language, the spoken aspect, had inevitably been ignored. We studied some American poems, which had images and metaphors I found hard to decipher. I could not speak the language or understand it very well. In order to improve my skills, and as a compromise to my strenuous objections at not pursuing more advanced studies toward fulfilling my dream of a professional career, I would be sent to school in Vermont, to a Catholic college for girls run by nuns. Considering it would give me an additional year of studying with some learning thrown in, and thus delaying the inevitable, away I went without resistance. In absolute terms, I was privileged, but given the world I belonged to, the upper-middle class, the notions of entitlement, the total ignorance of Marxist ideology in a society still adhering to the traditional hierarchy of the priest, the doctor, the lawyer, and the notary on top, then the merchants, and at the lowest level the farmers, the factory and domestic workers (this class system holding on until the 1960s) as a doctor's daughter it was unthinkable that I work in an office. Countless times, my sisters and I, in the course of doing so, were subjected to the following remarks: "Your father is a doctor, why then are you working here? I certainly wouldn't if *my* father was a doctor!" This hurt, since for at least two of us it had not been our choice. Further training toward nursing or teaching was out of the question, since years of tuition and lodgings were involved. It was too expensive, and our town did not offer the facilities.

My curriculum at this college consisted of typing, short-hand, statistics (a horror and disaster for me, since I didn't have a clue), English, and Spanish, which I enjoyed. I spent the first three months in total bewilderment, not understanding or speaking the language, and the full eight months in my familiar state of humiliating deprivation. The other American students, being from affluent families and able to spend whatever they wished, enrolled for the full four-year course. My fellow Canadians who were also there to learn English were from equally wealthy backgrounds. I was on a very strict stipend, and therefore isolated. My feelings of loneliness and dismay resurfaced. My parents were always oblivious to the fact that we were constantly the poorest financially and most neglected emotionally in whatever institution they saw fit to place us, although they maintained certain conventions in circumstances when their non-observance would have reflected badly on their social status. For instance, because it was traditional when a girl in our *milieu* turned sixteen to receive a fur coat, due to the very cold winters (the wearing of fur was always prominent in our country; after all, our economy had originally been based on the fur trade), my parents bought me a sheared beaver, which at least with regards to clothes put me on equal footing with the other Canadian girls. The American students who came from warmer climes and knew nothing about our customs looked upon us as complete aliens, given that we didn't dress as bobby-soxers, as they did. Jeans, which they called dungarees, were only worn by them for leisurely activities, but we were always more formally dressed than they were. Most of my compatriots at the college, not being as resilient as I was, did not last past the first semester. The culture shock was too severe. As it happened, they were the ones who had attended my convent. They went on to become nurses. Others remained and toughed it out. They had money, which made things easier. As for me, I knew if I left I would be returning to a loveless environment where I would continue in a commercial school and then on to a minor job, since my English was still far from being up to par. As the end of the year approached, I became more and more anguished.

A First Love

While attending the American institution, I had met a young man for whom I fell madly, as one would when one is in a state of helplessness: someone was paying attention to me. He was twenty-four, I, seventeen. He was not a college boy. Most likely I had met him in a bar, drinking a Tom Collins with my fellow female students, speaking French, an enticing trait to a more mature male. We used to neck in those days – *nice* girls didn't go any farther – for hours, in cars. Being employed, he owned one. I don't know now how the boys could stand it in those days. At the time, I was ignorant of male sexuality. He's the one who introduced me to putting my hand on a penis. I was shocked, but wanted to please and not appear a prude. I had never been close to the thing before, not having any brothers. I had caught glance of the male appendage only once before, when sitting in a row boat with my father in his gaping shorts, as he twisted his body to get the motor started with a rope. The sight had embarrassed me, and I quickly averted my eyes. I didn't like what I saw, that limp, purply, tubular flesh. This boyfriend's penis felt like a turkey's neck as he guided my fingers to achieve the up and down motion he sought. I recoiled at first, telling him I had never done that before. *Come on*, he said, *you're a French girl, this is your thing, don't play games with me*. He thought I was being coy. In those days — perhaps even now — English-speaking people thought all French people were sexual maniacs. He must have thought I was cute with my strong accent. He would make me repeat things in English I did not understand, and then he and his friends would laugh their heads off. I asked my American roommate what the meaning of "my pants are in the groove" was, and she acted offended, instructing reprovingly "Don't repeat that." She couldn't bring herself to explain. I didn't know *groove*. I looked in the dictionary, but the definition of that term did not seem to apply because I would not have expected someone to refer to female private parts so crudely and inanely in my presence. I just didn't get it. It was years before I realized fully the meaning of the phrase.

In any case, this young man understood that I never would go "all the way" and did not ask. I would not even let him touch my breasts, and he did not insist. Maybe he had another woman, but that would never have occurred to me at the time. We dated until I returned to my parents' home. We wrote back and forth, and I visited him once at his home. I don't think he came to see me. After a few months I received a letter saying he had met a girl and he would be getting married as his buddies were. That was the end of my first love affair and first steady dating.

I was devastated. I took it as abandonment, incapable of reasoning that since we lived in different countries, from such different backgrounds, it was inevitable and that the relationship could not survive. As I write these lines, I realize he was not even a nice man. I sobbed uncontrollably for hours, couldn't ingest any food for days, and my insomnia became more acute. For weeks, out of the blue, no matter who was present, I would have crying fits, making everyone very uncomfortable. An uncle proposed that we all go to a famous Chinese restaurant in Montreal. In gratitude for this act of compassion, I forced myself to eat and promptly vomited everything when I got home. My parents were at a loss. How could a break up with someone they deemed very ordinary produce such grief? Their indifference to their children's well-being precluded them from perceiving that my overreaction to the situation was but a symptom of something deeper and more serious: my feelings of hopelessness. I was desperate. I didn't want to live in my parents' house, depending on their goodwill, which was minimal. My siblings and I had always been considered a nuisance, but where to go without money? I had always lived a very sheltered existence, no street-smarts whatsoever.

The acute anguish which I had experienced for the first time during my last year in the convent had returned, but

I gradually regained control of my emotions in as much as I no longer displayed my distress. I attended a commercial school for a few more months, trying to improve my typing speed. I never became proficient at it, invariably hitting the wrong letters, no doubt due to my lack of coordination caused by the *essential tremors* which were worsened by my inner turmoil.

Two Cultures

I spent the last summer after college in the States with my mother and sisters at the cottage as usual. I had just turned 17 that June. The year was 1949. For two weeks in July, I participated in an exchange program with an English-speaking female student from another province. The purpose of the exchange was to familiarize ourselves with each other's language and culture by spending two weeks together in our respective homes. I went first. Peggy's father was a tobacco producer (nothing wrong with that in those days, everyone smoked earnestly). They lived in a small town on the shores of one of the Great Lakes. They were reasonably well-to-do. We had been matched according to lifestyles and social class, I imagine, so as to avoid too great a culture shock. Like me, she had just graduated, but was from a totally different environment, having always attended co-ed public schools. Although she was of ample proportions, which as is often the case had limited her dating, she was more accustomed to male behaviour than I was. Thus, she was able to introduce me to more boys I had ever encountered in my entire life.

Everyone was very curious of this French-Canadian girl, I being the first one they had met. As I've already mentioned,

Franco folks had kind of a sexy reputation then, the *ooh la la* thing. I was very popular with the boys, something I had never experienced before. I had always considered myself plain and unable to attract sexually. Father had consistently made fun of my Roman nose (same as his!), claimed I had too long a mouth, and a narrow forehead. He made me feel ugly, comparing me with my siblings, who were blessed with more regular features. To this day I remain self-conscious of my proboscis. I was mistaken, as I found out years later, in my seventies. I had been attending a Spanish class in the Caribbean, and the teacher, of African descent, stated in front of the whole class that he was nuts about my nose, that he would die for a nose like that. (He had asked another student, as an exercise in language, to describe my physical appearance.) His remarks about my looks, meant to be flattering, embarrassed me no end. Another male student in the class, in his thirties, observed the professor was hitting on me, hard, and sarcastically added that maybe I should remain on the island. No one suspected I was seventy-two!

On that student exchange program after graduation, one particular boy I dated, Aaron, who I felt I had more in common with than the others who were WASPs, was very offended when I asked him if he was "a Jew." My unfamiliarity with the intricacies of the English language had caused me to put it that way. I was not aware that a more gracious and accepted way of putting it would have been to use the word *Jewish* instead. I had never been acquainted with a person of that persuasion, and was intrigued by a creature who was neither Catholic nor Protestant, but of whose people I had heard much of before through my religious education, and more recently, the events of the Second World War. It was only four years since the end of that conflict, and the revelation of the horror had made me reflect. In my eyes, he was special. Disrespect was the last thing I wished to convey. When we parted that night, he had stated he'd "call me." He didn't, not the next day or the day after. I was puzzled and sad, not yet aware in those early days that men are wont to say that whether they mean it or not. I kept wondering what I had done wrong, pestering Peggy with questions. In the meantime, I dated others in turn. Being different, I was a sensation. Aaron was piqued. The word must have gone back to him that I liked him, or he figured out by himself that I was harmless, because after a few days he called and asked me out. What joy! I had pined for him. After that we saw each other quite often. In the evenings, Peggy would sit at home, always the gracious hostess, encouraging me to have a good time. Teenagers did not go out in groups in those days, unless they were double-dating, because whatever intimacy was sought had to take place in cars. I was out every night 'til the small hours, and got up very late the next day. My hosts never interfered, but I sensed the household was somewhat nonplussed by my social success. I had never felt so relaxed in my whole life. The tension which had been my lifelong companion was lifted. I was finally in a normal environment. I slept very well for the first time since I was a toddler.

After my two weeks amongst these very decent people, I went back home with Peggy for her stint of the exchange. It was our peculiar cottage life for her. There was a farm at the top of the hill owned by English-speaking folks where there were some teenagers our age, who my sisters and I mostly ignored. They ignored us, since we didn't speak each other's languages, but the animals, the barns, and activities such as hay-making aroused our excitement as city-dwellers. A new farmhand, Jim, who was thirty-two, took a shine to me, and of course Peggy could converse with him. This brought some kind of relief to her difficulties in understanding our family exchanges in rapid Quebec French. The version she had studied at school was more bookish, devoid of slang. She relished our excursions to the farm. Jim owned a pick-up truck, a vehicle she had used before, contrary to myself, who until then would not have been seen dead in one. We would meander up the hill nightly, Jim would take us for a ride, and inevitably we would end up at the inn that had just been built on the other side of the road from the farm. Within, there was a room with a bar, juke box and dance floor we called a *grill* in those days. Jim would invite us both in turn to do *slows* to the Big Band platters, all great swing music, and some jitterbugging. We drank beer, we smoked, and he paid for everything. It was a blast. Peggy was thrilled. She had never known such carousing, been so wicked. This place was no country club. You could easily run into disreputable characters. She surely went back home with the impression that in spite of our strict religion (fish on Fridays), we were a very permissible society. It's just that our family was different. That was the luck of the draw for her.

In Peggy's small town, the youngsters she frequented were offspring of her parents' friends and acquaintances. It was the same in our circles, actually, but in our family's case, the out-of-town schools and the cottages on fishable lakes for Father's sake had isolated us from our peers. Both she and I were exhilarated at stepping out like this: I, because it made me feel important to have someone spend money on me and desire me; she, because for once she was popular, never mind being taken to a nightclub and associating with a farmhand, something she would not have been allowed to do with an employee on her father's tobacco plantation. She happily disregarded those moments when I was able to steal some "necking" sessions with Jim, moments when she had to seriously practice her French with my siblings who could not speak English, and who were flattered and pleased to entertain this older foreign girl whom they could sense was somewhat shocked and titillated by the free-for-all.

I never allowed Jim to go too far, and to his credit, if he tried, he didn't insist. We weren't monitored. My mother was aware of this man's presence in my life — thanks to my sisters' tattling — and made disapproving noises. He was, after all, almost twice my age, "beneath our station," but she certainly did not suspect that we were sort of making out. She figured Peggy and I served as each other's chaperones. This sort of activity outside of engagement or marriage was unknown to her. She would not have indulged in forbidden, sinful acts (to be mentioned in the confessional) when she was that age, or ever, for that matter. I found Jim more interesting than boys my age. I think he'd been in the army. He always respected my limits, and he realized he was on dangerous grounds: fooling around with a doctor's daughter who lived in a summer cottage right on a lake known for its elite dwellers. But he was also flattered, not realizing that if I wanted some semblance of romance I really had no choice but to accept his advances. I probably acted as if I was doing him a favor, quite aware of my social standing in those days. That was my last summer at my parents' cottage. Once all my sisters started working for a living, Father sold it for a pittance. It is easily worth

$500,000 now. We regret not inheriting it. We go for rides, drive by, and reminisce. It is such a beautiful spot.

When summer was over I found a job as a secretary at one of the town's car dealers. My salary about $20 a week, if that. When Father asked me to pay board, I took it very badly. As far as I was concerned, it was adding insult to injury: not only had I been denied further education, but at seventeen, in my posh family home, I was expected to share my meager wages. It struck me as the height of insensitiveness to my feelings of having been gypped. The offense was so great, I flew in a great rage which they had never seen, and told Mother in no uncertain terms what I thought. I could not have discussed it with Father. He would have become very angry at being contradicted, and I was terrified of him. Mother succeeded in making him accept a minimal sum so he wouldn't lose face. Handing over what he had originally asked for would have left me penniless, and thus once again without control whatsoever over my existence – we never had an allowance — not to speak of the indignity.

PART TWO

A First Career

<u>Earning a Living</u>

Secretary was a fancy term for the work I did in my new job. *Receptionist* was more like it, taking down and typing the occasional letter as well. Lucky for me: I was such a poor typist. A car dealership is a very lively place (kind of rough too, in the parts department in the back). Almost everyone owned at least one car fifty-seven years ago. I was not bored, and my depression was receding somewhat. The clients were only male, and in the 1950s overtly admiring the female figure was not frowned upon. I basked in the attention. I dated a mechanic a couple of times. He would have liked to make out, but he did not dare make a move, and I was not forthcoming, conscious of our respective places in the social order. But our dates were talked about and must have come to Father's ears. He was on the board of the local paper, so after a while, he mentioned he could get me a job there, at the very bottom of the ladder. I accepted the offer. Again, my salary was a joke. I was assigned to newspaper clipping and reporting on weddings and funerals. I had the feeling my co-workers, besides ogling my figure, were making fun of me. One of them, as it happened, had been one of the twin altar-boys in the convent, but not the one I fancied. He asked me for a date. I declined. I intensely disliked his nasal voice. As it turned out, he became a famous media personality, extremely talented, full of shit and very wealthy. In one television interview, he claimed having sported a shaved head when he was a teenager, maverick that he was, the only one in the fifties looking like that. I immediately phoned my sister: "G.F. is on TV making up stories about his past. Men didn't have long hair in those days, never mind shaving their heads. What a liar. As if he needed that to make himself interesting."

There was another reporter at the paper who years later, at my father's funeral, confided upon expressing his condolences that he had been in love with me at the time I worked there. This co-worker certainly had not let on at the time. I was hardly aware of his existence, but I remembered him. I was moved.

After a few weeks as a junior journalist, still feeling ill at ease in that environment, I quit. I was too young and screwed up to know you have to give it a chance. Father was not happy with my decision, and I don't blame him. It was the first time he had done anything for me, but I had absolutely no appreciation of how far such work could take me. I had never imagined myself in a writing career due to my lack of self-esteem, self-confidence, and fear of ridicule. Being an emotional basket case at the time, I was entirely incapable of making an informed decision about my future. I was still imbued with the desire to attend university. Being a reporter — the "media" concept was still in its infancy — was not an exalted occupation in those days. I had never heard of columnists. Journalism was a trade, not a profession, and it didn't feel to me like a respectable endeavour. In my small town, no one was revered in that field.

Romance

About that time I started dating a saxophone player who, like my former American boyfriend, was seven years older than me. His being a musician meant that on important nights, Saturdays and Sundays, he had to play in his band, and I had to sit there in whatever club and listen while everyone else around was dancing their hearts out. I resented that. So, immature me, after a few months broke up with him. I regretted that achingly. That feeling of abandonment engulfed me again, although the abandonment was my own doing. Perhaps I thought he would beg me to take him back. He didn't. I didn't know how to make up, full of silly pride, nevertheless miserable. It turned out he had his own problems: he fell ill with pneumonia (which was diagnosed as TB) and was eventually sent to a sanatorium where he was treated for at least a couple of years. Once declared "cured," he no longer had the breath to play his instrument. It was very sad. I don't know if he took it up again. I lost track of him. New medication came out for that disease and it was almost eradicated. Now it's back. Father said, sardonically, "You're lucky you didn't catch it."

Years later, while dealing with cancer, one of the scans I underwent showed I had healed scarring on the lungs. There had been TB in my maternal grandmother's family. I may already have been immune when I necked with my musician boyfriend, and I certainly would be now, unless exposed to a new virulent strain.

At the same time this was going on, I was being courted by a Greek boy named Spyro, whose family owned a restaurant next to Father's pharmacy. We went out for a while before I left to work in Montreal. Apparently, I was the love of his life. He married a woman from his own community, became an alcoholic, and later committed suicide.

Monkey Business

During those months, I lived alone with Father in our city home while Mother stayed at the cottage with my siblings. Something happened one night which interfered with my already troubled sleep for the rest of the summer. Father and I both came home around 1 a.m., he from his social club, quite intoxicated, and I from a date with Spyro. In the early fifties the style in women's clothes featuring the cone-shaped bras was very revealing, especially if you were as endowed as I was, with an hourglass figure. Father, leering grotesquely, made a gesture as if to put his arm around my back and slurred something in my ear about my breasts. It reminded me at the time of the Mickey Spillane detective story I had been reading, *I the Jury* (my very first work in English, in fact). It mentioned firm breasts pointing like torpedoes. I had picked up the paperback where it had been dropped or discarded on the ground and decided to have a go at it. It was easy language to understand, being very basic. I moved away from Father, giving him a stern look. *Don't even think about it!* Being drunk, his will was not strong. He would have collapsed at the slightest push. He did not insist. In the recesses of his stupor he knew this was a bad idea, otherwise he could have become very angry, as was his wont when contradicted under the influence. A glimmer of decency rising from the depths of his wantonness spared me. It never happened again, but I was nervous being alone in the house at night, sleeping fitfully, feeling very weary the next day, unable to type adequately (a task which, in my case because of the *tremors,* depended on a serene state of mind).

Some evenings I would accompany Father to the local ballgames – the reason why baseball is the only spectator sport I understand. The minor league team featured some Puerto Rican and Dominican athletes. One evening as we were leaving the stadium, we came upon some groupies who were waiting for the black players whom they viewed as stars (they being so exotic in our exclusively white environment). Father pointed to one of the young women and asked me if I didn't think she looked like we could be sisters. This question really startled and puzzled me. Why would he say something like that, considering that her behaviour was, in my opinion, deplorable?

This incident increased my anxiety. I experienced the same sort of feeling some months later, when going from house to house, collecting for the United Way – an activity I abhorred given my shyness and rejection complex, but had volunteered for out of civic duty. A woman in a flat just down the street from our home told me with a knowing smile I could not decipher at the time (which made me feel very uneasy) that she knew my father very, very, very well. The other women present were nodding in agreement, derisive smiles on their faces. Upon inquiring with Mother about the matter, I was told that she would not know, for in that place lived loose women. This was news to me, mysterious; after all, we lived in a better section of town inhabited only by families. The only whorehouse I knew of was on Main Street. There had always lived a girl younger than me there, who attended the second convent where I boarded, a creature with the exotic name of Magella who later turned out to be one of my uncle's, the dentist, mistresses.

Mother's response had been so unemotional and off the cuff that I did not even suspect what was going on. I found out right after Father died, but as he lay exposed in his coffin I missed something which would have been a shock to me, although it would have allowed me to put two and two together regarding the young woman at the baseball game. According to my sisters, Mother asked her brothers to stand guard at the door of the funeral parlor so as to bar the entrance to Father's long-time mistress, who indeed came to pay her respects. She was thus prevented from doing so. (I did not notice any of this.)

When I finally learned the truth, I found it didn't affect me anymore. I was fifteen years older and married with my own life and problems. Although Father was a monster in many ways, I still loved him. He was honest to a fault, incorruptible. Outside his carousing and medical practice, he had devoted his time to public life and was very involved in civic matters. He had been a co-founder of the famous local zoo, and the first president of the town hospital (the nuns who ran the establishment respected him and spoiled him with gifts of homemade *sucre à la crème)*. He certainly was bigger than life, probably suffering from undiagnosed hyperactivity, which he self-medicated with alcohol and pills. Due to his notoriety, carrying his name made us feel special. I had stopped caring for my mother when she had demonstrated her determination that my fate would not be better than hers.

Husbands' adultery was commonplace amongst my mother's relatives and their peers in general. My uncle with the girlfriend from the whorehouse managed to squander his wife's fortune with his wenching. In those days, my aunt had no recourse: being Catholics, if her husband wished to remain married, she was stuck. This aunt had a twin sister, also wed to a dentist, who used her inherited money to gamble, seduced their teenage babysitter (perhaps it was the other way around), and took up with her. That couple did divorce (such a scandal!) and he married the sitter. The sitter happens to be the sister of another uncle's wife. All in the family. The girl remains to this day ostracized by her relatives. That first uncle died years ago from lung cancer — he refused therapy and continued smoking for three months after his diagnosis — and the other dentist is still alive, in his nineties, still married to the babysitter. The twin wives are unfortunately much the poorer, the considerable wealth left by their parents dilapidated by their spouses.

I learned that the place on Main Street was a house of ill-repute when hearing of my uncles' arguments to convince my aunts not to oppose Grandfather's remarriage one year after Grandmother's death. He had been seen frequenting the brothel at that address. Grandfather was almost seventy, and in those days, that was old. He did indeed remarry, a woman in her fifties, to my aunts' disapproval. This step-mother was not in as good a shape as expected. The poor woman died before Grandfather after having an eye operation which left her demented and locked up. He lived alone after that until the age of ninety-four. The last years were very difficult for him. He was not used to solitude. My youngest aunt used to go and bathe him; managing the bathtub was a problem. He wouldn't eat, wishing to die. The uncles were not involved. It was a daughter's duty.

Grandmama's Death

Grandpapa's last years were sad but poetic justice, since Grandmother, who had given birth to sixteen children, died alone, while, as usual, her husband was spending the evening at the Knights of Columbus, playing cards with his cronies. I remember that night very well: I had been out with my dog, Bijou, and stopped to chat with some young man I knew. I was ready to walk back home when I noticed Bijou had disappeared. I looked everywhere for him, calling his name, but couldn't find him. Then I remembered that fire engines had been out on the street with their sirens blaring some time earlier. Bijou had always been terrified of that sound. The only place nearby where he would have taken refuge was my grandparents' house. Worried, I hurried there, rang the bell, and found to my great surprise that Grandmother had let him in. She never liked dogs, not even ours. I was even more amazed that she invited me in "to talk with her for a little while." She seemed cowed and somewhat grateful to see me. She was not fond of my sisters and I, had always found us rambunctious, and the way Mother dressed us irritated her. She was an elegant lady, while we were frumpy. She probably also projected onto us the hostile feelings she harbored toward Father, who certainly did not support us the way a doctor was expected to. Father hated her. When he had started courting Mother, she had warned her daughter not to get involved with him, because she felt he drank too much. Mother ignored her advice, to everyone's later great regret. Mother, rightly so, thought Father was more intelligent and interesting than her other beaux.

The night Grandmother died we were all asleep. When the phone rang, Grandfather wanted to speak to Father. Upon his return from his club, he had found Grandmama unconscious. She had been suffering from angina. When Father got there, she was already gone. I figured that when she had asked me to sit with her earlier in the evening, she had a premonition of her own demise. It was the only time she had ever been pleasant with me. I remember the events as if it happened yesterday.

The circumstances of Grandmother's passing had a lot to do with my resolve not to have many children, and later becoming a feminist. She was a talented woman with exquisite taste when it came to fashion, and had sewed all of her five daughters' clothes, who were reputed to be the best-dressed girls in town. In another era, she could have had career as a designer. She certainly would have been very smart had she not been in the clutches of her faith and religiosity, which kept her ignorant and bigoted. I never saw her but cranky, no doubt frustrated, confined as she was in her role as housewife and mother, even though they were well-off. Every summer, once the children were grown, my grandparents toured the Gaspé region, and every winter spent six months in Florida. Grandmama's retirement did not last very long. She was sixty-two when she died.

It's a Jungle Out There

After I broke up with my musician, my life became a desert, socially and romantically. There didn't seem to be any reasonable husband material around. Father had mentioned some of his younger professional colleagues found me attractive, but as they appeared to me more or less cut of the same cloth as he, although flattered, I demurred. I quit working for the newspaper. I shouldn't have, but at the age of eighteen and in my anguished emotional state I was not in a condition to make responsible decisions concerning my future. It was decided I would go live in the big city. Through family connections, employment for me as a secretary (the term *administrative assistant* had not been invented yet) was found in a French import/export firm where my office skills were at the disposal of several men. It could have been interesting, but because of my faulty typing, I was scared witless. I disguised my nervousness by humming constantly while I was working, not noticing I was the only one doing so. I saw people smile at me. It did not occur to me that this was not appropriate behaviour, and that they were laughing at me. I was also still innocent about the dangers of being unknown. This was not an environment where my family name and status meant anything. I was just another female employee at the bottom of the hierarchy, since I was the last one hired.

At that point, having become aware of my attractiveness after years of thinking myself unable to charm, I was still exhilarated by the idea of it. In true fifties style, I flaunted my physical endowments — not my cleavage, but my shape. This was bound to send signals, unbeknownst to me, that I was "available." And, as someone remarked some thirty years later, as I was deploring the effects of aging on my figure, "Well, your face is not exactly a disaster." It was a scenario right out of the television series *Mad Men* (this was the fifties, after all). One of my bosses, who was middle-aged, asked me out to dinner. I suspected he was married but I had never been asked out to dinner by a man before, especially in a fancy restaurant in the big city. I had no idea what that implied. I was flattered and, always the *gourmet*, only feeling slightly guilty that he was not single, I accepted the invitation. He picked me up in his expensive car and took me to an establishment in the suburbs, a location totally unknown to me (the better not to be seen, I guessed later). He had reserved a private room which made me uneasy. He seemed to be well-known to the staff, who no doubt knew very well what he was up to: about to consume virgin flesh. He advised me on what to pick on the menu. We drank the best wine, which he made sure was flowing in my glass. Little did he know about my capacity to imbibe. I have never lost control long after my drinking companions are practically under the table. When he figured I was ripe for picking toward the end of the meal, his face flushed, he put his hand on my breast. *Whoa!* I backed up in my chair. None of that business with me! He turned livid with rage, so sure I knew the code, would play the game. He was probably ready to fuck me right then and there. I feared he would hurt me in his frustration (which I did not understand), that he would take me by force in his fury. Did he not know you don't touch good girls? Perhaps he would stalk away after having his way with me and leave me there in the middle of nowhere. He must have read terror in my face, because he slowly calmed down and took me home in silence. The next time I ran into him at work, he was friendly and even joked about the incident. He would not hold it against me. He was a gentleman after all. But I had learned a lesson. I found out that you can't arouse a man without being willing to deliver. It was not fair, although it was, paradoxically, in those restrictive times, common practice.

I was ashamed, not because of what today would be considered sexual harassment at work, but because I had been so naïve. It brought home the point that I was not as sophisticated as I thought when it came to the ways of the world. I was probably viewed as a country bumpkin at the office. At the same time, my employer being a French firm, the atmosphere was Old World, and there was nothing casual or relaxed about it. Although I was perpetually filled with anxiety, probably fuelled by the question of what was going to happen to me, I did not act humble as I should have, considering that I was a female nobody. I did not know how to act subservient. I was not happy, but in my ignorance I blamed it on this particular place of employment. I started looking for another job. I answered an ad for secretarial work at a paint company, and had a successful interview, probably because of being bilingual. I also had a letter of recommendation from my former employer (although certainly not for my typing speed, which remained abysmal). There was nothing refined about this place, and I disliked it immediately, but I had to earn a living and prove that I had made the right decision in quitting my other job.

The person who had secured employment for me at the import/export business was very offended that I had not stayed there. She claimed they had done her a favour by hiring me, which is likely, since I had very little experience. Father was furious for the same reason. None of those considerations had entered my mind. I had no idea how things work in the jungle out there. Little had I realized that I might be falling from the frying pan into the fire. The young Anglo managers in the various departments at this new company ogled me. Since I did not have a boyfriend, and I would have liked to have one, I didn't mind. One day, a couple of them proposed that the three of us go for a ride during lunch hour in a convertible belonging to one of them. I thought it strange they did not propose going out to eat. I was not sure what I was doing there as we set out, and tried to make innocuous conversation. Maybe they expected me to suggest we have sex during the break or arrange it for sometime later. After all, I was a "French girl," "stacked," and a lowly office worker, apt to be accommodating. They weren't saying anything, as if expecting something from me, and looking grimmer and grimmer as the hour passed. I was confused. I sensed they were displeased. I still didn't know the score, how to deal with men. I knew I had not provoked them.

Sometime after that, my boss called me in his office, and said I had no business correcting his spelling and grammar after he dictated a letter. Who did I think I was? And besides, my typing was too slow. He fired me. I was filled with dismay by the unfairness of it. Had I not been taught in business school to render a perfect letter when it was submitted for the boss's signature? I thought I had done my duty, that he would be pleased to be sending out impeccable documents, considering he was practically illiterate. Of course, if you were as crassly ignorant as he was, you wouldn't know that. Thus I learned that you have to gauge people who have power over you in order to survive. Never show them up.

Horny Relatives

At this time I was still living with the family of a paternal aunt whose home was located in a classy borough of the big city. My uncle was an insurance salesman, a former classical singer, whom the Depression had forced to secure a steadier occupation. They were in dire straits, but my aunt, being a consummate snob (as acknowledged by Father and her two other sisters), insisted they live in that part of town, that their three sons attend university, and that the daughter take some courses there. She was not intended to achieve a liberal profession but to catch a suitable husband. She did: someone ugly as sin who became a university professor, famous in his field, and ended up heading some government commission. My cousin herself later recovered from breast cancer, the occurrence of which was proof in my mind that she was not fundamentally happy in her marriage. A lot of doctors do not agree with this theory, that a void or suppressed emotional stress in a woman's life causes the disease. I beg to differ. I've met too many widowers, always very authoritarian buggers, whose wives died of breast cancer.

My aunt's and uncle's best friends were a doctor and his wife whose daughter ran away to Paris with a world-famous painter when he was still unknown. What a scandal, especially for Auntie and Uncle, who were strict, moralizing Catholics. At the time, two of their sons lived with them.

The oldest, a lawyer, was already married (to Auntie's great disappointment) to a woman of lower middle-class background and, a greater sin, with no family money. This cousin, who thank God I did not see very often, was tall, dark, and handsome, grandiloquent and patronizing. With the arrogance of youth I could not understand why he had chosen someone who was so ordinary-looking. She was a lovely person, though, very kind to me. It might have been the rebel in him: my aunt was constantly riding her sons about making a "good marriage." She was endlessly conniving to find the most profitable match for them.

My second-oldest cousin was a resident doctor at one of the local hospitals, and therefore mostly away from his parents' home. He was the black sheep of that family: not very good-looking, cocky, funny, and lecherous. He would regale me with stories about fucking all the nurses, such willing creatures, bent as they were on catching a doctor husband. In those days, all this *libertinage* shocked me. I had not expected nurses to be loose women. He tried his luck with me, nothing subtle about it, and mocked me when I spurned his advances. For him, the fact that we were close blood-relations clearly did not enter into the picture, whereas I had had it drilled in my subconscious by my religious upbringing that you did not fool around with first cousins. Literature has taught me otherwise, but at the time, I was not a specialist. None of the books the Church had allowed me to read covered the subject. Years later at a relative's wedding, as we were dancing, he confided he had tried to read one of the novels of the author I was working on for my Ph.D. thesis, and confessed to finding it difficult. I was amazed that he would tackle such a work, indeed, that he read books, but then he added he had always been in love with me. He had been drinking but I believed him. His laboring on a difficult novel I was interested in was proof enough for me that he cared (football being his main interest outside his profession). Of course, when I mentioned this incident to a sister of mine, she sniffed, "He loves all women." I should have replied, "Has he ever told you he loves *you*?"

He was married to a woman his mother had found for him. He had always professed, not discreetly, that what he was looking for was a rich wife. This woman was indeed from a wealthy mercantile family, educated in the best schools, refined and high-maintenance looking. What was she doing with my raunchy cousin? It was rumored he regularly cheated on her. She remained married to him because he was a doctor, from a more prestigious background than her own. She herself was not a nurse, a status which would not have been good enough for Auntie. Besides, from what I gathered at the time, doctors did not have much respect for nurses. Perhaps that's why so many of them do marry nurses, the same reason business men marry their secretaries: it keeps them feeling superior.

Why didn't I become a nurse? Had I not been brought up in a medical environment? Taking care of sick people is a vocation. It requires a certain mentality I did not have, and I did not see doctors as gods, was not consumed with the desire of marrying one. My cousin's wife was always very nice to me when I saw her at weddings or funerals. I was surprised she remembered me. He had a big mouth. He might have told her I was a nice girl. He died of pancreatic cancer in his fifties. We all missed him. He was bigger than life, like Father in many ways. Also, being a pediatrician in the city's children's hospital, we had all called upon him at one time or other when our kids were sick. He was always happy to oblige.

Little did he know that when I spurned him, his younger brother was also hitting on me, and to my great shame, I was reciprocating. Not all the way, naturally, I would not allow it. He certainly would have taken advantage, had it been a possibility. He was also tall, dark, and handsome like the eldest, and very smooth. Whenever we found ourselves alone in the house, we would start necking passionately. I felt very guilty and would report it dutifully in the confessional. But it did not stop me. Somehow, my aunt and uncle got wind of what was going on. Maybe they could simply feel the sexual tension in the air. Without warning, or having any discussion with me in that respect, I found myself ostracized, and my gorgeous cousin disappeared (in as much as we never found ourselves alone in the house again). I was not told of family functions; he was introduced to another female cousin on my maternal side, not related to him, and started dating her. All of this was done behind my back. I was being punished, the evil female who had led the poor, helpless male into temptation. When I finally understood what was going on, I was very hurt. I felt betrayed. Of course, our illicit, libidinous conduct was, in my aunt's and uncle's minds, a mortal sin, and true to original lore, I was deemed the temptress.

This cousin, although attending university, did not know what he wanted to do with his life, to his parents' dismay. It was found out later that he was bipolar. I was with him in a car much later on, as he was driving us to visit his mother in the hospital — no one knew what was wrong with her — in one of his manic phases. It was an ailment I knew nothing about. He talked non-stop, jumping from one subject to another. I thought, *The guy is losing it, perhaps from the stress of seeing his mother so ill.* He too had married a rich girl found by Auntie, according to his own wishes. He finally committed suicide, and then I was relieved of the humiliation they had inflicted upon me.

Meeting the One

In the meantime, I had found employment as private secretary to the branch manager of a British insurance company. When he interviewed me, he casually inquired about my skills, never had me tested, and hired me on the spot after ten minutes. The fact that I was bilingual and quite literate in English was a main factor in my favor, I believe. He had been transferred from Ontario to oversee this Quebec branch. The man was hardly ever in his office, and he enjoyed drawn out lunch hours. His position did not seem to require actual hands-on work. Outside of the few letters he dictated and which I typed with all the time in the world, and some filing, he did not ask much of me. I was not impressed by his diligence, but obviously nothing more was expected of him. Still, I felt contemptuous of what I felt was his laziness. Because I was the boss's personal secretary, nobody else in the place could touch me, so outside the fact that it was boring, it was an ideal job for a digitally handicapped person like me. It is one of the ironies of life that years later, as I sat in court as a municipal judge in the Ontario town where I ended up living with my husband, his son appeared before me as a defense lawyer. I suspected the relation when I heard his name (one you could not forget because it was unusual in that in vernacular German, it was the word for male genitalia). They were very self-conscious of their name, of which I had learned the meaning from snickering office co-workers way back when. I inquired of the son if his father had worked in Montreal during the fifties and informed him that I had been his secretary. I asked him if he would please convey my regards. Obsequious as all lawyers are toward magistrates, he feigned interest and said he would relay this message to his now-retired father. I doubt that he bothered. His father would have been in his early eighties by then, and must have seen many secretaries come and go during his career.

I was supporting myself, but I had not a single friend. Auntie had introduced me to some young women of her acquaintance, but considering that they were all either going to university or living a very comfortable life at the home of well-to-do parents, dabbling in the arts until they found husbands, with social circles well established since childhood, they had no incentive in pursuing a relationship with someone with whom they had nothing in common. They were busy; what did I have to offer them in return? Meeting me had been a chore imposed by their mother at my aunt's request. They were being polite, and I could feel all this. It made me even more despondent and awkward. Maybe if I had been mousy they would have taken pity on me. I was not wise enough to act humble and charming in those days, although I certainly suffered from a vast inferiority complex exacerbated by my circumstances. I wondered how Auntie explained my situation. Snobbish as she was, she must have mentioned that her brother, my father, was a doctor. I did not fit. My cousins never brought any of their friends or *confreres* home, and without girlfriends I would never have ventured by myself in a nightclub. I was very lonely. If someone had told me that one day I would be the fussy one, very picky about choosing friends, and sought after, I would never have believed it. I was still what my environment had made me, and marriage seemed the only solution to my problems, although finding an acceptable man was in itself the biggest problem.

One day I went to my neighbourhood bank, and there, lo and behold, was a girl from my graduation class, a day-student at the convent who had lived across the street from the school. She had been very friendly with the famous twins, one of whom I had refused to date when working at my hometown's newspaper. She was toiling as a teller. Her family was not well-to-do, and there were numerous children. Her small town provided no decent employment for people with our genteel education, and like me, she could not afford university, hence how she ended up where I ran into her. She proposed we go on a double-date. She was going out with an Anglo who would bring a friend for me. I said sure, although I was not overly fond of her. All I knew about her was that the girls in her family enjoyed quite a lot of freedom. They had a reputation. She had sort of a sloppy demeanor. But I jumped at the chance of an outing, even if it was a blind date. We made arrangements. They were to pick me up at my place. The bell rang, and my aunt let me answer since I was expecting them, and there at the bottom of the stairs were two young men grinning at me and saying my name. One looked like a Greek god, albeit Celtic, and the other one was a runt. My heart sank. I just knew the runt was for me. My friend stepped up and introduced them. Oh miracle! the good-looking one was for me.

That's how I met my husband. We were both nineteen. I suspected later that in the first months of our relationship, my friend sampled him. I shall call him Speedy. He was very handsome, extremely bright, and exceedingly charming, but crazy. He was already employed, but drank every day after work in some tavern or other, for hours. For the purpose of our dating, Speedy had the use of his father's car. In those days you could drink and drive with impunity, and he did, insanely, recklessly, cars being the ultimate *macho* symbol. His driving added to the relative lawlessness of the Montreal driving scene. When Mother rode with him for the first time from the city to our hometown, she was so terrified by the experience she shook for two days afterward. On later occasions, Speedy took this into consideration and tempered his madness to accommodate her. That was something he never did with me. In the early days I did not voice my fear and disapproval of his manoeuvers behind the wheel, but throughout our marriage his manner of driving caused me great stress, compounded by the fact that in spite of my pleas for moderation, my feelings were, as in other circumstances, being blithely ignored. I was later satisfyingly vindicated in that regard, when I learned that one of our daughters-in-law refused to step in a car driven by him.

Speedy was not like any other boy I had ever met. He was streetwise and incredibly resourceful, very, very bright. He introduced me to a world I had never heard of. He frequented jazz clubs, knew about reefers, and was familiar with prostitutes. He drank a lot, but that was not shocking to me, considering my father's habit. We went out dancing

Annemarie Duparc

several nights a week or he would visit with me at home, which was the custom then. My aunt and uncle disapproved entirely of him, first because he was an Anglo who spoke our language as he had heard it on the factory floor, and second because he worked in a plant. He did not have a profession. He had started working right after high school and therefore was not worthy of our family, although they themselves treated me like dirt. His only saving grace in their eyes was that he was Catholic. When he called on me, they felt it was their duty to chaperone us by angling a mirror in the hall in such a way that it would show what we were doing in the living room. By their standards, young people were not supposed to engage in amorous activity before marriage. The automobile was by necessity our means of getting intimate. We were both in our late teens with raging hormones. We indulged in long necking sessions — no intercourse.

One time, we were parked in an isolated wooded area, making out like mad when I heard what I thought was a branch breaking. I stiffened. We could be attacked, I could be raped, the car stolen. Speedy scoffed. I was imagining things. Suddenly, the face of a scruffy youth with a salacious grin appeared at my window. He was standing on the sideboard and grabbed my arm through the open window. I screamed. Another one appeared on the driver's side. Where a different individual would have been paralyzed with fear, as I was, the fighter in Speedy reacted instantly. In a few seconds he had turned on the ignition, put the pedal to the floor, and we were out of there, crashing through the woods, the intruders flying off the car. I felt he saved our lives, and I was full of admiration. I told him I would never neck in a car again. We had been told to move on by the police before, which had mortified me, but this was it. After that, I started thinking about getting a place of my own.

An American Cousin

After her sons had definitely left home, Auntie had one unused bedroom. She decided to increase her income by giving refuge to an elderly distant cousin named Eldred. He was an American by birth who had been a gold prospector in California and had ended up in the Canadian West. He was a bachelor and still in possession of the money he had accumulated over the years. We were his only relatives. He came east to visit and Auntie offered him the opportunity to spend the remainder of his days in her home as a boarder, her eyes on the inheritance. This manoeuvre was observed by her brother and sisters, who knew very well what she was up to.

Indeed, when he died, the inheritance was equally divided between them, and my father received his portion of it. Had my aunt not looked after him, God only knows what would have happened to the money. The fortune would have disappeared in the hands of lawyers and local sharks, as happened more recently with another American relative, a successful gentleman also from California whom we knew vaguely of, but of whom, as it turned out, we were also heirs. There was a quirk in the will, however: only the daughters of our grandfather stood to inherit, and therefore, my father was excluded. We, as his surviving daughters, would not be involved. The money would be divided between our surviving first cousins. There was not such a big amount to be shared by eight people, but there were lands and properties down there. The eldest of the cousins, the lawyer (now a retired judge in his seventies), made the trip to California to look into it but came back empty-handed. He had not been able to establish in the eyes of those who now held the properties that the Canadian cousins were the beneficiaries of the estate. It was too far away, and at his age and in his physical condition, he didn't have the fight in him. The results, had they won, were not worth the cost of litigation.

Eldred, of course, was not polished, and my aunt felt nothing but contempt for him. She was using him. He was not allowed to eat his meals with us, as she did not approve of his table manners. He was a sloppy eater, being more or less senile. I don't think she even served him the same food as us. He probably should have been in a home for the elderly, needing specialized care, which she more or less provided, but not graciously. The way she treated him upset me.

Then my life in that place became unbearable. Eldred started coming into my room in the middle of the night. I would wake up and he'd be standing there at the foot of my bed. I would shout for him to go away, but he was obstinate as old people can be, whose minds cannot analyze what they are doing. I told Auntie. She talked to him, but it didn't register. He kept it up, and I lost my sleep, knowing very well what was on his feeble mind. I could have knocked him over if he had tried to act out his impulses, but night after night? I knew my aunt would never relinquish that source of income, so this gave me the excuse to look for another place to live. She appeared vexed, but I knew she understood my position very well. My parents were annoyed, but what did they care? My father especially knew how strict my uncle was, and that it would have been hell living with him.

The Engagement

In those days, I was making $32.75 a week. In my lowly functions, I was paid by cash in a brown envelope. It never occurred to me to figure out how much that came to a year. Office workers did not think in those terms. The flat I found from a newspaper ad was in an apartment building downtown. It was a real dump. Now I also had to feed myself. I was miserable, but I had had no choice. I was poor and knew no one I could share lodgings with. The only advantage was that my boyfriend and I could now be together without being spied on, and neck to our heart's content. We also went out and drank a lot. I started taking sleeping pills. With all the upheavals in my life, insomnia had now taken a firm hold of me. I had to work during the day in order to support myself. Since tranquilizers and anti-depressants did not exist for ordinary people like me, the only remedy was medication of the opiate variety, which left me groggy and more depressed during the day. My relationship with Speedy was stormy; often I would not see him on the weekends, his reason being that he had to accompany his family to their summer shack. I resented that tremendously.

He had one particular shady friend who would bring as gifts to his parents items he had lifted from stores. Speedy thought nothing of this. I was shocked that he wasn't shocked, and that he consorted with a thief. This was so far removed from my way of life that I kept asking myself what I was doing with this guy. Later, in the sixties, it turned out a lot of students indulged in this practice, but when I was nineteen, still imbued with all my original values, it was something I wanted no part of. I gave Speedy an ultimatum:

you stop associating with this person or I'll stop seeing you. He agreed. I never heard of the thief's exploits again. If he did disappear from my boyfriend's life, I had no way of knowing. Later on this man was knifed to death in an illegal gambling joint, and I triumphantly pointed out to my then-husband how justified I had been in barring him from his life.

Speedy's environment was white trash, a concept I was not aware of in the fifties. I was fully confident that with his smarts he would rise above his background and had a brilliant future ahead of him. I kept telling him so. He was really into me, and into the idea of taking out a doctor's daughter, which I exploited, so that was sufficient incentive to make him stick by me, although he was somewhat drawn back to people of his ilk. His mother had earmarked a girl for him to marry. His family (that is, the women, his mother and sister) totally disapproved of me and contemptuously gave me the cold shoulder. Ironically, this was discrimination in reverse, given the difference in our backgrounds and the fact Speedy had been fully accepted by my parents. I surmised that it was my being French-Canadian they objected to. His father, being a rascal like my own, must have had girlfriends of my tribe over the years. In their mind, I had to be a slut. Nevertheless, after many scenes from the females in Speedy's household, we became engaged.

Speedy bought me a diamond from some wholesale merchant. What bothered me was not the size of the stone but the design. It was bow-like with chips, very old-fashioned looking, and I would have preferred a solitaire. I was annoyed that we had not chosen it together, given the fact that he didn't have much money and therefore his choice would have been limited to crummy designs. But I understood that he wanted to surprise me and pretended I was delighted. I never liked the ring and could sense a lack of admiration in anyone I showed it to. I dutifully wore it for thirty-five years. One day I spotted a new jewelry store in the neighbourhood where the owner designed rings and saw one I very much admired in the store window. I brought him my diamond and asked him to make me a new one in that model, which was very modern and unusual. I was complimented on it. One daughter-in-law inquired if it was a new ring, and I finally told the story of how I had never liked my engagement ring. I had long ago known the marriage itself was a disaster, and longed for my husband to admit it. *Wow*, was my son's reaction, *and you never said anything.* I told him I did not want to hurt his father's feelings. My husband said he never suspected anything. Of course he didn't, he only saw what he wanted to see.

After our engagement, I would occasionally be invited for dinner at my future in-laws' dingy and soot-covered first floor apartment. Speedy's father was the building superintendent. What struck me the most was that they served soft drinks with the meals. I remembered my mother's words: "Only poor people drink those." At our house the children drank milk and my parents drank tea, or wine on special occasions. I myself have never departed from that custom for health reasons. His father would make passes at me, and I would push him away with a pained smile. His wife would exclaim, "Mac, stop that immediately, leave her alone!" Not a hint of indignation in her voice, just feigned disgust, as if talking to a spoiled child, as if this gross familiarity was not at all inappropriate behaviour, yet she was extremely religious and puritanical. They watched over their own daughter's virtue like hawks and were extremely strict with her, hence her deep resentment of Speedy. Being male, he could come and go as he pleased, and he ruled the roost. My father-in-law's lewdness was even more shocking to me because he was cold sober. The man didn't drink. I was miserably aware I did not belong there, but I felt I had no alternative in my dire circumstances.

On some weekends we piled in the family car, which was driven by Speedy's father with total disregard for others on the road. Upon my whispering about it in my fiancé's ear, he surreptitiously explained to me that it was his father's way of looking for a fist fight, which he often provoked, and always won, being very strong. He was establishing his *macho* superiority. The man went around looking for action. We were going to the family shack in the country. His sister was excluded, but Junior was present. He was only in his early teens and was mostly ignored by everyone. Speedy's mother informed me that becoming pregnant with him was the biggest surprise of her life. She was fond of repeating that at the least provocation. I gathered from that remark, and so must have Junior, that she had not been crazy about the idea of having a third child when she already had a boy and a girl. He was a nice kid. Not tough like his brother, whom he emulated career-wise and even surpassed. He was always looking for thrills like skiing straight down a suicidal hill or flying his own plane. He came to a tragic and rather early end in an African country where he was doing business. He was said to have drowned, a victim of a heart attack, but the whole incident remains dubious. It is thought he might have been a spy.

The summer shack had two small bedrooms, just big enough to go around a double bed, and one main room where the cooking and eating took place. They would let me have one room to myself, but in the mornings Speedy would invariably join me in bed and grope me to my immense embarrassment. The others were so close by, the walls so thin. I thought his parents should have objected. Our behaviour highly improper. Speedy was never reprimanded about anything, which would enrage his sister, but it did not occur to her to blame it on the double standard. Appropriately, she married an ex-Jesuit. They were a very religious couple, had three children of their own, and then out of Christian charity adopted the daughter of friends when the mother died giving birth to the child. They were extremely strict with their brood when it came to anything even remotely approaching sex. My sister-in-law's husband died at the age of forty-five from all the pills he had to take for a very painful form of arthritis.

While he was alive, the children had not been allowed sleepovers at friends' houses in case some monkey business would take place. After their father's demise, the oldest son, who was by now a strapping teenager, started sexually abusing his two younger sisters. The mother was out earning a living during the day; did she ever suspect anything, as is often the case in father/daughter incest? If she did, she would have vehemently rejected the idea. She was too goodie-goodie. Sanctimony is fertile ground for deviance. They came to terms with the problem when the adopted sister, upon reaching adulthood, denounced her brother.

Those sessions in bed with my fiancé (a word which in those days did not mean "you might as well be married") made me very tense. I would freeze, and I could not digest my breakfast. We had been engaged for a year and a half and Speedy was giving no sign that he wanted to actually marry.

69

I believe by now his parents were mainly opposed because they needed the additional income his board provided. Although we were wonderfully sexually matched, I was not enchanted anymore. I threw the engagement ring back at him and told him we were finished if he did not make up his mind and if we did not fix a wedding date.

I did not feel secure in the furnished bed-sit where I was living. There had been an incident where one of my neighbours, a man, had started howling in the middle of the day. I figured in my fevered imagination he was an addict in need of a fix, in the throes of withdrawal. Finally another man appeared, carrying what seemed to be a doctor's bag. He didn't bother closing the neighbour's door entirely. I peeked, and saw him retrieve a needle and inject the howling one, who soon calmed down. I was shocked and frightened, because drug addiction was not so common then, and I could not imagine living so close to it. I called the police, who came, listened to me, and asked what proof I had that an illegal transaction had taken place. Just seeing a needle was no evidence, and the man was quiet now, the fixer gone. The incident made me feel like a fool, made me realize my helplessness. Another neighbour, a single man who was either retired or on social insurance, never went out of his apartment and quietly drank all day. The beer was delivered. The sight of such loneliness devastated me. That aspect of the human condition was also new to me.

My parents came to visit in my new lodgings. I don't think either of them had imagined such wretched surroundings. Of course, Father had often ministered to poor people in our town, but it looks worse in the big city. I heard him say, not believing my ears, "Our daughter should not have to live in a place like this." I believed he was about to offer to help me out financially. "It's her choice," replied Mother. "She does not want to live at home, so she has to suffer the consequences." Her tone was spiteful. *Once again, I thought, my own mother does not care.* Did she resent the fact that I had had the guts to flee the family drama where she played the victim so convincingly and I could be witness to her suffering? Of the four sisters, only the one who was Mother's unique object of affection stayed at our parents' home for years, thriving on her own rage against Father and affirming Mother's martyrdom. She only came to work in the city when the youngest of us graduated from secondary school and in turn had to find employment. This latter one would not consider living with our parents any longer than I had, and for the same reasons. The two of them together found a decent place to live and did not have to experience the same unfortunate conditions, such as being practically penniless and alone, as I had.

On this visit to my seedy lodgings, Father (being as usual in his cups) could easily have been swayed one way or the other. In this case, it was easier for him to go along with Mother's pronouncement. His good intentions did not materialize into a concrete gesture. So that was that. I looked for another place and found a more acceptable one, again from an ad in the paper, which I shared with two other young women, but with a bedroom of my own. This apartment also featured cockroaches a plenty, but by this point I was beyond caring. It also prepared me for similar encounters with those ubiquitous insects in my later life, such as in the graduate library when I was studying for my doctorate. In my new home we were all in the same boat money-wise, but the other two girls did not have steady boyfriends. One of them struck me as pretty loose, coming home one night with torn panties. While I was living there before my marriage, disenchanted with my relationship with my fiancé who drank too much, I had a romantic relationship with a fellow worker. Physically, of course, it never went any farther than any other I had ever had, but this gent being British was polished compared to Speedy, better educated, and of a background more compatible with mine. I broke up with him after a couple of months because he was Protestant, and in those days very much a foreigner to me. I was still very much bound by my culture. I have memories of happy moments with him. Speedy was not sensitive enough to my moods to notice anything.

The Wedding

The wedding was set for mid-October. It was to be a semi-*grand marriage*: mostly relatives and close friends of the bride's and groom's parents' were invited, as well as some of the betrotheds' best friends. The list was arrived at by the bride's mother, given that, as was the custom, the bride's father assumed all expenses. In my case, a certain amount was allotted for the event, what my parents said they could afford. They had never borrowed money in their entire lives, except for a mortgage when they built their house. It simply was not done, and I never questioned that philosophy, which I share to this day. Mother bickered a lot about how much it was costing, making me feel guilty, but I didn't have a cent to contribute. I suggested that instead of hiring an official photographer we ask a cousin who was a keen amateur. It never occurred to me to forsake the big wedding and take the amount instead, as did one sister when she got married. All the girls I knew from school had

had the traditional ceremony, and perhaps because I was marrying "down" compared to them I wanted to at least be like them in that superficial aspect.

I asked this same sister (who was the second eldest) to be my maid of honour. She refused, claiming she was not about to spend any money on that. I was very hurt. There were to be no bridesmaids either. Speedy, who really did not have any presentable friends, asked my uncle, the dentist, to be his best man because it was not the tradition in the Anglo world to have his father act as such. All those deviations from propriety added to my ambivalence about the wisdom of this step I was about to take. My parents seemed satisfied. For Father it was two daughters gone, two to go. In addition, as in the case of our elder half-sister's husband, Father was very happy with Speedy as a son-in-law, who, as was customary, had duly asked for my hand in marriage. At last, he had someone he could drink and go fishing with, and they got along famously. This, after all, was the first adult male besides himself around the house, given his first daughter lived miles away, never visited, and was very happy in the bosom of her husband's family. Speedy was bright, and very handy to have around, as he could fix anything. And he was so charming with Mother, which was something she was not used to.

The invitations were sent. Perhaps my persistence in pursuing this disastrous undertaking that was my union with Speedy was ultimately an unconscious attempt to please my parents, who had never shown any gratification in my existence. I had quit my job in the big city and was residing at home. I was becoming more and more anguished, sleepless. I certainly would have done things differently had I been the autonomous, self-assured individual I am today. In my heart I knew I was doing the wrong thing, but I needed a home of my own and thought I would eventually find in marriage both the material and emotional comfort I had never known. Still, I felt I was heading for disaster. The night before the wedding came a very bad omen: Hurricane Hazel raged all around us, and it turned out to be one of the most destructive storms ever in our area. I was sharing a room with my youngest sister, who recently told me I had confided something very disturbing to her on the eve of my wedding: I did not want to get married, a revelation which had left her very distressed, wondering what to do. What could she do? What a burden to carry.

The next day was beautiful and extremely warm for that time of year. Everything went according to plan: champagne flowed, speeches were made by important people. As weddings go, it was a great success, and I remember the event itself fondly. A distant relative told me afterward that as I was kneeling down facing the altar next to the groom, our backs turned to the guests, she had spotted one of my feet shaking furiously during the whole ceremony. You must have been nervous, she told me. If she only knew.

We were going to New York for our honeymoon. Since Speedy did not have a car of his own, he had been offered by one of his male "acquaintances" I had previously never heard of a splendid vintage sports car which would take us to the Big Apple. I had my doubts: another one of Speedy's schemes. Everyone gathered around to admire it. We certainly looked very sporty and hip as we took off in that roadster, but as I feared, it conked out before we reached the American border. I didn't think it was funny. After many phone calls and much persuasion, his father agreed to deliver his car to us, and take care of the antique.

By that time I was in a state of silent panic. What had I got myself into? We motored on to New York, stayed in an unglamorous hotel (all we could afford), and gorged ourselves in a famous Italian restaurant, which made me sick since I was still too tense to digest properly.

Speedy was a very good lover. He obviously had had practice. I was very receptive. Sexually, our union was a great success. I knew this was not given to everyone. That was the advantage of being with someone who had been around, and probably why we stayed together for so long. I was determined to succeed where my mother had failed.

A Home of Her Own

The other aspects of the marriage were not so remarkable. We moved into an apartment above one of Speedy's colleagues, who was also a newlywed. His bride, a plump young woman, was wise enough to continue working, whereas I, who was driven by the compulsion of righting my parents' marriage, chose to be the perfect fifties wife. I stayed home, dedicating myself to my husband's needs and keeping house. I was bored stiff. For lack of funds, we had little furniture, and I thought it was cheap-looking. Speedy's father, as part of our wedding present, had painted the apartment for us in colours of my choice, which I thought would be sophisticated and stunning, but the combination of which in the kitchen was jarring. It was too advanced for the times, and the ordinary folks who would drop in on us would snigger. As for the few acquaintances and relatives of my own who would visit, I knew they were surprised at how lacking we were materially. Hippie-style living had not been invented yet. If you did not have all the latest appliances and many furnishings, you were either poor or an artist. I soon stopped inviting anyone over, although in my unemployed state, I was very isolated and lonely.

I spent considerable time washing and ironing my husband's white shirts, five a week, to perfection. It was actually a task I enjoyed, and Speedy would boast about my homemaking skills. Even my mother-in-law had to compliment me on them. Ironing white shirts was a chore she had never had to do, her spouse being a building superintendent, and even if she had had to, it would have been shoddily performed. "Second-best is good enough" was her motto. If you don't aim too high, you'll not be disappointed. She reveled in repeating that mantra, her unconscious way of riling me, sensing I was striving to be the all-round perfect wife, a notion which seemed foreign to her. Given that all she ever had to say about her husband, Mac, was that he was a good provider, she probably felt that she did not owe him anything more. She certainly was right at that. In any case, she most likely sensed that her son would never have the opportunity to say to me that he preferred his mother's way of performing any household task.

When I started living with him, I was shocked at the way he never wrung his facecloths and left them dripping from the towel bar onto the bathroom floor. It was such a far cry from what the nuns and my own mother had taught me. On the other hand, having never seen my mother cleaning the house, it had never occurred to me before I married that someone would have to do it if I acquired a home of my own. Soon after moving into our apartment, looking at the toilet bowl, I realized that since we could not afford a cleaning woman, I was the one who was responsible for keeping our abode spotless, without fail. I was still very much plagued by the sense of strict discipline instilled in me by the nuns. Not a pleasant prospect. This situation was permanent. I had found my man, and no longer was I living in temporary digs. Fortunately, I liked cooking even more than ironing, and although I lacked experience (because Mother had never let us help her), I soon became good at it. Speedy often joked that I should open a restaurant.

One of my mother-in-law's favorite left-handed compliments for me was that I had such "good legs," meaning they were fat. She herself was obese with piano legs. In fact, when I wore high heels (which was all the time before I had children), I was blessed with very shapely gams. One day a biker who had seen me put gas in the car at a highway station started following me on the road. I thought something was wrong, and was also somewhat scared. At a point where we had to stop, he motioned for me to lower my window. I was not at all reassured. "I just wanted to say you have the most beautiful legs in the world" was his remark. What a relief. When I shared this with one sibling she sniffed it was just a pick-up line, implying that this biker thought I was the kind to go with him.

I now had a permanent, decent shelter, but I was still very unhappy for lack of money of my own and a social network. It occurred to me that the only kind of work that would suit me and bring me satisfaction (given that a university-acquired career was out of the question) was to do translating work from English to French, although at that time there was not much demand for such a service and therefore no official studies in that field and no diploma. Besides, I had no connections and did not know how to go about getting such work. Perhaps being always tired from having to take sleeping pills for my insomnia, my listlessness aggravated by marital friction and idleness, I lacked initiative and imagination when it came to venturing into the unknown. I was self-defeatingly paralyzed by the predicament of not belonging where I had ended up.

Speedy, to whom I had always touted my desire to be a perfect homemaker and lover, was enchanted with that state of affairs. He was not about to delve into what I was getting out of our life in common. Having lived through the hell of my parents' marriage, and no doubt because Father showed no discrimination in hating his daughters equally, whereas Mother at least loved one of us and had demonstrated that one wasn't me, I by now blamed my mother entirely for the dysfunction in our family. I had decided and was determined to do better. Such is the naiveté and arrogance of being a twenty-year-old. I was convinced I could manage my life so as to put things right, to redress the parental errors which had ruined my early life. I chose a drinker and a sadist for a husband. My childhood circumstances had to be reprised in order to be corrected. The patterns imprinted on our psyche during our youth are so reassuringly familiar that no matter how vicious, they do not appear lethal.

Unlike my mother, who could fall asleep before my father came home in the middle of the night, I waited anxiously for my spouse to return in the small hours, inevitably loaded to the gills on numerous occasions. I couldn't get over the number of "retirement dinners" he felt obliged to attend. All wonderful occasions for getting soused, since he had considerably curbed his drinking sessions right after work, now having sex to look forward to at home. When I compared notes with other wives whose husbands had attended the same company events, it was clear that Speedy was always the last one to leave, holding forth until everyone had gone home. Contrary to those other wives, I would lie there, miserably watching the hours slip by, waiting for his return. When one's sleep is fragile, insomnia is guaranteed for the whole night when triggered in such a way. It aggravated my depressed state the next day. This habit of Speedy's continued even when there were babies. I couldn't understand what was so enthralling about those dinners. His fellow workers considered them a chore and often skipped them. Once he had put in an appearance, why did he not just leave and come home? Speedy was the embodiment of what was known as a "company man," but at the time I did not understand the dynamics of the situation, the attraction of the booze and male company.

We couldn't talk, and what I said did not matter. It was as if he couldn't hear anything that didn't suit him. Perhaps since I had vowed to him that I would be the best of wives, he believed that should be enough for me, that it was owed to him. I felt so very much alone. His demands with regards to his marital rights were incessant, but since he never failed to satisfy me, and Father had so often, in a rage, complained of Mother's lack of interest in that regard, I felt compelled to grant my spouse's every wish (although I did object to anything approaching anal intercourse, which was, in those days, certainly unheard of by women like me; I found the mere idea of it terrifying, the pain!). I had a vague notion that's what homosexuals did. Very weird; doesn't it hurt frightfully? I knew nothing of Vaseline or lubricants, as the subject had never come up in my sheltered life. The few times I did refuse Speedy's advances, mostly when I was upset by his being inebriated after he had promised sobriety, he would throw a tantrum and bully me for the rest of the day.

Before the sexual revolution, women's carnal entitlement did not exist. I myself never used sex as a way of getting my way with my husband, but that's how the game has been played since time immemorial. I believe it was Germaine Greer who wrote that marriage is glorified prostitution, which are my feelings exactly. That's why I never used sexual favors for extorting material benefits from my husband. I suppose it could be argued that getting decent shelter, which I could not afford living on my own, was that kind of transaction, but at least I enjoyed the sex. After twenty years, when feminism was well implanted, I came to view forced copulating, devoid of pleasure for the woman, performed as a duty, as rape. In the early years, the fact that I reached climax whenever we had intercourse did not mean I wanted to do it all the time, but I was driven by the obsession that he would never have to look somewhere else for his sexual needs. It worked.

Pregnancy

The pill had not been invented yet. Our means of contraception was the rhythm method, the only one allowed by the Church. I was convinced that if I observed the rules the beast gnawing inside me, my unhappiness, would disappear and I would finally be like everyone else. I was not ready to have a child. I felt that we couldn't afford it, and that we should enjoy a bit of financial ease before incurring further expenses. In my family, parenthood had always been vilified by deeds, if not in words. Motherhood was much less exalted due to the risk of having numerous children one couldn't cope with. I accidentally became pregnant after three years. I noticed something was different when one day the smell of eggs made me sick. I can't remember how my condition was confirmed. We did not have a family doctor in the city and I had always relied on Father for medical advice. I should have put myself under the care of an obstetrician, but it did not occur to me. Our relative poverty might have had something to do with it. Health insurance did not exist yet. No doubt my cousin, the pediatrician, could have given me references for finding care during my pregnancy, but I wasn't keen on having anything to do with him, or of being reminded of my life among those particular relatives. I had morning sickness twenty-four hours a day, retching dry so hard that I would get a pain in my temples as if I had burst a vein. The nausea abated somewhat after the first three months, but was replaced by something I had never heard of regarding my condition: profusely salivating to the point of having to constantly spit out the excess, and persistent, extreme drowsiness. Worrisome and very unpleasant. Being very narrow of hips, I carried in front in the shape of a football, and I couldn't see my feet in the end.

The last month brought back some energy, and I was looking forward to the great event, bustling about, getting everything ready. I went home to my parents, and the baby was delivered by Father (to his great reluctance), but I had insisted, for he had done it thousands of time. The real reason was that having been financially and emotionally deprived all my life, I would have felt guilty spending money for my own medical needs. I was not worth it. Speedy, pals with Father, and whose people were strong, healthy, and poor (doctors being a luxury), thought the arrangement dandy. The baby boy weighed eight and one-half pounds at birth, after a long labor, coming out with the help of forceps, ripping my vulva. I had been put to sleep for that first one. There were no other alternatives to ease the ordeal in those days, certainly not in a country hospital.

Post-Partum Depression

When I took my newborn home, I found that I could not fall back asleep between feedings. I was not nursing, and there was no La Leche League then. Mother had always warned us not to nurse: if you had a lot of milk, the heaviness in the breasts is a killer, and you will always be exhausted. She was very well-endowed, as was I, and she had nursed all four of us, believing that doing so would prevent a new pregnancy. It had not worked. Not nursing when my breasts were full of milk produced excruciating pain the few days I was in the hospital. Why did they not pump me? Perhaps such a procedure was not known yet. In any case, between preparing the formula, looking after all the other baby's needs on a rigid schedule (you did not feed on demand), making sure I was doing the right thing, and trying to run the household, I did not find time to wash, comb my hair, or get dressed. Exhausted from the lack of sleep, I lived a nightmare. There was no joy at all. I was overtaken by a sense of total hopelessness, made worse by not knowing what was happening. It is now known as post-partum depression and there is medication for it.

I looked at my body. My old bras did not fit anymore, and my breasts had changed shape, sagging. I would observe other new mothers and wonder why they weren't miserable like me. I cried, wishing the baby would die so I could get some rest. I did not want to take more sleeping pills than usual, so I would not be too groggy to look after my child.

I talked to my parents. We moved to my hometown, and Mother looked after the baby for a while. I was ashamed. I could not explain why I was not like other mothers and I was worried about what people thought. Nobody understood why I couldn't just fall asleep like everybody else. They could not fathom my distress.

My parents had the bright idea to send me to a priest who had the reputation of having "advanced ideas" for the times, and who mused my husband was probably too demanding regarding the frequency of sex in the circumstances, and perhaps in general, which was entirely accurate. True to his calling, this priest also advised the best way to improve my situation would be to have another baby. Immediately. That did it. I snapped. The Church had it in for women. It was not where I would ever find help. Nobody close was going to help me. I would have to depend on myself. I became an atheist that day.

One Flew over the Cuckoo's Nest

I expressed my frustration and rage and pointed out the incredible stupidity of the priest's suggestion to Father, who did not openly agree with me, but decided to send me to one of his colleagues, a psychiatrist in another town, who was very proud of his new method of dealing with depression: electric shocks. I was hospitalized. This guy reeked of liquor – that was his bond with Father. He would give me a needle and then turn on the current after applying some kind of contraption to my head. The discharge would jolt me one foot in the air. I was still conscious, not at all relaxed, which would explain why later when X-rays were taken after a car accident it was discovered that I had ancient fractures in my lower back. After two such treatments (which gave me an inkling of what the death penalty in the electric chair was like), I categorically refused to submit anymore.

A girlfriend of mine who lived in that city came to visit me in the hospital. As I was explaining to her what had brought me there, joking, putting on a good face as usual, she exclaimed, "But you don't look sick. What do you mean you can't sleep?" Of course I was looking well. In the hospital, I was taken care of and I could sleep at least five hours without interruption. My back was sore, but I was entitled to pain killers. Even when drowsy, I wasn't expected to do anything but lie there. Pretending I was cured I returned back home, still in the full grip of despair.

My condition had made me aware of Freudian theories and psychiatry in general, which was in all its glory, not yet competing with chemicals for treatment of the mentally or emotionally disturbed. I was convinced that it would be the solution to my problems. Although I was able to catch a few hours of sleep, the baby no longer waking up in the middle of the night, I was still filled with the same anguish I had always known. I was gripped with anxiety to the point of distraction: I would go to the supermarket, stand in front of the meat display without being able to make a choice, panic engulfing me, as if it was the most momentous life and death decision. I started seeing another psychiatrist (I don't think we called them psychotherapists in those days) who thought I would be cured by a stay in a private clinic for rehabilitation of wealthy alcoholics and emotionally-impaired people. Since my experience with the priest, whose asinine advice would have further destroyed me if I had followed it, I had opted for looking after my own interests if I wanted to survive. I informed my parents that they would have to look after the child while I went away for treatment of a condition they were responsible for, quoting Freud on disorders caused by events during one's childhood. Utter nonsense, he didn't believe any of that shit, sputtered Father in a rage. "The psychiatrist says I have to be hospitalized," I stated, "otherwise I want to leave my husband." That would have been worse in their opinion, I surmise. What to do with me if I became single? They did like their grandchild, they were normal in that way, and so they agreed.

I entered the clinic where dwelled patients suffering from all kinds of psychological ailments. I remember three of them specifically. One was a mother like me who simply could not cope with a young son who today would be diagnosed as suffering from hyperactivity and attention deficit disorder. She had become a nervous wreck. Another patient, also a woman, was actually demented, in her sixties, and who might have suffered from Alzheimer's. In her madness, she kept repeating, so logically, "I don't go to church anymore, their prayers always say the same thing. Very boring." The third person was a *Chartreux* monk, from a monastery I had never heard of somewhere in the province. I never really understood why he was a patient there. He was not depressed. I seem to remember there was a problem with him following the rules of his order. We became very close. I suppose there was sexual attraction. We enjoyed each other's company greatly, but we were warned about it, spending too much time together.

Patients suffering from depression were treated with shock therapy, in anticipation of which they shivered in terror. They couldn't remember much afterward. I wasn't convinced the benefits would last. I was spared those since they had already been tried with me. For my case, insulin therapy was prescribed. I'm not sure how it works. I was given a big injection and then be hit by a rush of inexpressible anxiety, characterized by the feeling of literally falling into an abyss, like that heart jump in an elevator, except that instead of lasting seconds it endured for one hour, accompanied by extreme sweating. Anxiety had been my lot in various degrees since I was a child, but with the insulin I literally had the feeling of dropping off a cliff. After two such treatments, I told them I was no longer depressed, I dreaded them so. I was discharged. I could have stayed there forever with my friend the *Chartreux* monk, yet at the same time I longed so desperately to find fulfillment with my little family. I resumed looking after the baby, who, as I had dreamed of, was very good looking with curly hair and a lovely smile, making me proud.

Feeding him with a spoon was a real chore for me. In my weariness I had little patience, and he felt it. He was never very hungry and didn't gain much weight, compounding my worriment. What was wrong with me? Why couldn't I be like other young women who slept well and appeared to be quite relaxed, combining motherhood and housekeeping? I did not know that when you suffer from depression after giving birth, you have to be treated appropriately. Electric shock and insulin treatments do not apply.

Speedy and I did what other couples did for entertainment. We went to movies, to dances with people we knew from his work, visited my family and his, but I did not feel at ease with the other wives because I couldn't confide in them. They wouldn't have understood, nobody would have. I put up a good front. I had not lost my figure. I was lively. The gals probably envied my looks; their men clearly were attracted.

The boss and his wife, who came from old money, oozed class and therefore were more sophisticated than Speedy's co-workers and spouses. They accepted me as one of their own. They appreciated my background, and I felt very much at ease with them. They had tons of kids, and a butler. She remarked, as I mentioned my hours of labour, that when her time came she would drop the babies like a cat, with hardly any contractions or pain, the delivery almost a surprise. She also felt heavenly during pregnancy. No wonder they had so many kids. It was a far cry from myself, who suffered during the whole nine months. How I envied her, but still, I liked her very much. .

Speedy continued his heavy drinking every chance he got. We were invited to a wedding for a college friend of mine in a small town in an area I had never visited. Her father had been Premier of the province for a short while, and the whole thing was very posh. The ceremony was outside in a tent, with champagne galore and anything else you wished to drink. A certain dashing boat captain, spouse of the bride's best friend, and who was drinking rum, offered some to Speedy, who, having already imbibed tons of alcohol, should have refused. He could never mix drinks. But he had to match the other one glass for glass. I tried to stop him, but he was too far gone to heed me. He never paid attention when it came to booze anyway. When the captain had enough, he left. By that time, Speedy was white as a sheet, looking very poorly indeed. We walked toward the mansion where I was hoping we would find a bathroom very quickly, but as we crossed a living room, he spotted a sofa, a period piece, very fancy, covered in damask, and simply and unexpectedly lay down on it, a perfect stranger in that house where the guests had been kept outside. I was embarrassed to tears, terrified he would vomit on the Persian rug and furniture. I pleaded with him to get up, but he didn't hear me. He looked as if he was passed out. Someone came by and asked me who that was on the sofa. I had to explain he was not feeling well. A security guard arrived and told him he had to leave the house. I was mortified. I knew nobody else there had behaved like that. The guard helped me walk him to the car and place him in the back seat. I wanted to get out of there as fast as I could, but I was also in a rage that I couldn't say my goodbyes to my friends without bringing their attention to the fact that I was married to someone who did not know how to behave. I was humiliated, and it wouldn't be the last time.

Would I be so sensitive had Father not been such a shameless drunk? But I had another problem: I had not driven in years. The only time I had used my father's car I had had an accident, and I had never tried again, considering the torrent of verbal abuse I had been subjected to on that unfortunate occasion. I did not know my way back to the city either, but I had no choice. I was too embarrassed to seek help. I summoned my courage and my memory, got the car going, lurching ahead (it was not an automatic) and fortunately traveled on country roads with few other cars. Suddenly, Speedy sat up and asked me to stop. Thinking he wished to pee or throw up and rid himself of the poison, I let him walk across a field of high cornstalks where he disappeared from view. I waited for him to come back, but it was not happening. I went to find him and there he was, sleeping on the ground. I woke him up and engaged in another session of imploring him to get up and back into the car. At that moment, again I was faced with the questions: What am I doing with this guy? Why is this happening to me? How did I get in such an untenable position? He finally yielded to my arguments that we could not spend the night there and agreed to come back to the car. I eventually found my way home. It was a memorably bad experience.

Thanks to his boss appreciating my husband's talents, said boss not being ambitious and not fearing competition from his up-and-coming employee, Speedy was promoted. He fully deserved it. We moved to a bigger flat on the second floor of a duplex. There was an extra bedroom and soon I started sleeping there. Speedy snored sonorously and that disturbed my already fragile sleep. There is no doubt I was still in the throes of depression. I did not enjoy playing with my child, and always being so weary, I found it tedious. There was no daycare available and you did not bring your children everywhere with you when you had to or wanted to go out. For nighttime, there were the occasional babysitters. I had no family near. Once he stopped sleeping in the afternoons, my son was also bored, so I decided to put him in his harness and tie it to the balcony railing downstairs where he could play with some toys on the grass and watch the action on the street, especially the fire engines coming in and out of the station at the next corner. He found that very exciting. Too exciting. One day I heard the sound of screeching tires as a vehicle down below came to a forced and sudden halt. I ran downstairs in a panic and saw my little one in the middle of the street, surrounded by puzzled firefighters who wondered where he had come from, where he belonged. He had managed to wriggle out of his harness and had started toward the fire station. I found him unharmed and unaware of the commotion, but the feeling of what might have happened, of having been negligent, of guilt that engulfed me is still with me today as I write these lines. I'm afraid at the time I scolded him for not staying put, but I hugged him and kept him close to me for the whole day. He was only two. Of course he wanted to go look at the fire trucks. After that, in spite of our tight budget, I hired a young girl to take him to the park every day. The time to myself also eased the tension.

Expecting Again

Two years after the birth of our first child I started thinking it was my duty to have another one. Why was I so consumed with the notion of doing the right thing? I became pregnant as soon as we stopped using condoms. No longer under the thrall of the Church, I had stopped using the rhythm method. The nausea started again, but at least I wasn't constantly salivating, as with my first pregnancy. Instead my nose was blocked and I started talking as if I had a head cold. People remarked on it. It was worse when I lied down. I could not breathe except through my mouth. I was unable to sleep. What was this new predicament making my life more difficult? I did not think of it as a medical problem, believing it would pass. The condition stayed with me for 30 years, alleviated by the use of nose drops at night. At one point I consulted a doctor who specialized in allergies (it was not a specific specialty yet) and after analyzing some tests made on my skin, he declared that it was probably due to dust, whatever type of particles floating in the air, and perhaps endo-something, which I understood to mean that I was allergic to some substance inside my own body. It didn't seem avoidable. This condition of my nose immediately blocking the minute I lied down has disappeared for a few years now, although it starts running whenever I ingest the same kind of foods which are responsible for my irritable colon syndrome. It remains a mystery to me why pregnancy was so hard on me.

A Child's Pain

When I was five months into carrying my second child, S., my first, P., contracted a rare and terrible ailment called the Stephen Johnson Syndrome in reaction to taking penicillin. Certain membranes in his body (his scalp, inside his mouth, his ears, his palms, and the soles of his feet) became covered with oozing sores, which caused him excruciating pain. He was just a child, and he could not understand. I could not bear to see him like that, and I had no idea what was wrong with him. I immediately called my cousin, the pediatrician, who had him admitted to the children's hospital. After a couple of days he was diagnosed with this syndrome, which could have been fatal. He was to remain at the hospital for three weeks. It was the middle of winter. I would call a taxi and visit him every day. In those days there were no provisions for parents sleeping in hospitals with their sick children. P. would scream and hold on to me when it was time for me to leave. I was torn apart. He did not know what was happening, wrenched away from his home, in pain, given needles, amongst strangers. I was sick with the anguish of knowing what he was going through.

One day there was a snow storm, no cab to be had. Determined to go, I asked the landlord (who I happened to run into downstairs) if he would take me to the hospital on his way home. "That's out of my way," he said. I explained I couldn't get a cab because of the weather, that my child was dying in the hospital and I had to go see him. "Where's your husband? Why should I take you?" I begged him in tears. He finally agreed. It dawned on me then that indeed Speedy should be by my side during these taxing moments, but he was carrying on with his life as if nothing had happened, never mentioned at work what had befallen us, just as his boss was never told when I was operated on for cancer. They certainly would have allowed for his taking some time off to deal with his son's illness. I assume Speedy was afraid of appearing "sensitive," not *macho* enough if he made such a request. The landlord did take me to the hospital, shaking his head, reluctantly, adding shame and sorrow at being so treated by my husband to my worry about P. The child was never the same after that, moving (or rather, not moving) in a sort of daze which infuriated his teachers in his first years of school. They couldn't get him to get dressed in winter time when class was over and it was time to go home. His hair, which had been curly, went straight. When he came home from the hospital, he was on cortisone, which left him constantly famished. He became almost obese until I protested to the doctor, who stopped the medication. One good thing that came out of his stay in the hospital was that he started talking a mile a minute in complete sentences, having had to share a room with other kids. He had been behind in that regard, perhaps confused due to the use of two languages at home.

Full Motherhood

S. was born in late spring. He was the smallest of the three, but in his case labour had to be induced, and I was very much afraid that he might have suffered a lack of oxygen in the process of delivery, but he was fine. He was a beautiful baby with strawberry blond hair and blue eyes. P. was less enchanted by his arrival. At one point he said to me, "We don't want to throw the baby out the window, do we?" Shortly after his birth, we moved to the suburbs where we had a house built in a development under construction. We had chosen our own model, different from those offered by the contractor. When we moved there, we were the only house on the street. There were no sidewalks or paved roads yet. P. could play outside and run around to his heart's content. I was very lonely there. I did not have my own car and there was no bus service.

Even when other people started moving in the other houses eventually built on our street, I felt alienated from the other women because of the tiredness and depression, unique to me, and unexplainable. I would take the children for a walk, S. in his carriage, P. by my side. One day a delivery truck ran over a dog right in front of us. I had seen it coming but had not reacted fast enough due to my state of habitual exhaustion, practically paralyzed. I felt terrible, sick about it. One of my neighbours had seen the incident from her window. She came out screaming at me. How could I have let a poor animal get killed? How could I have not warned the driver? There was no way I could explain my condition. I was racked with shame and guilt. She was in a rage, as if I had wanted the poor creature to die. It was not her dog, but it seemed she was taking it personally. Later

I found an underlying cause for her fury. At the inevitable neighbourhood parties I was a magnet for the male spouses, which no doubt their wives resented. Physically speaking, I was in all my glory, and vivacious, well informed on most matters.

I never let on how I felt. There was no point. The only times I've ever looked sick in my adult life was after the laparoscopy for removal of my ovaries in 1974 (I hardly ate during that stay in hospital, the food being inedible, adding to the sense of hopelessness, and as usual I was devoid of a support system) and the other instance my misery showed is when I broke my leg at the age of seventy-four. Hopping around on the other leg for weeks was an absolute killer.

An Unwanted Pregnancy

I became pregnant for the third time when S. was only seven months old. I did not want another child. I was not ready. I was still too fragile to start another round of totally sleepless nights. I didn't think I could survive, but abortion was not even considered. It was unthinkable. I raged against my fate as a woman. There was nothing to distract me from my fear and isolation. At one point I asked my mother if she would be with me after the birth to give me a hand in the first couple of weeks. She refused. Her excuse was that she had to prepare for her darling daughter's wedding, which was to take place the next spring. My child was due at the end of November! Her darling had a small, intimate wedding, and there was little to organize. Mother must have figured she had done enough for me with my firstborn. The thought of dealing with two rambunctious youngsters was no doubt daunting, and she was not about to make the effort. My wellbeing had never meant much to her.

Why I should have felt so rejected I don't know, I should have expected it, but it added to my despair. It was like being at the bottom of a black hole I couldn't climb out of. I would have liked someone to take over and say "don't worry, we'll find you someone to take things in hand after your baby's birth until you're back on your feet," but there was no one. And all along, the guilt for not measuring up.

That September was very hot. I had sewn a pregnancy outfit, corduroy for the winter, but with no sleeves, a jumper I could wear in the heat. I felt if I did things like that, womanly activities, I might be rewarded by becoming normal. The baby inside me was growing bigger and bigger, and I could no longer see my feet. The food I ingested would come back up for lack of room around my waist. It was impossible to find a comfortable position in bed. The labour lasted twenty-four hours, with severe contractions all along. In spite of the birth opening being strategically cut by the doctor to facilitate the birth, my vulva was torn every which way and had to be sewn with consequences I would suffer with for the rest of my life. R. weighed eleven pounds, eight ounces. I have very narrow hips. My fear of being put to sleep had prevented me from accepting anesthesia. I felt every minute of it. At that time it was the thing to witness delivery with your own eyes. My sister-in-law had told me with much pride and haughtiness she had been able to do so with the help of a mirror. Her shape was the opposite of my own, flat on top, wide below the hips, so pregnancy no problem. It made her high. Caesarians were reserved for certain cases, which were very rare.

When our third son was born, he had a form of eczema between his little fingers (toes), at the crook of his elbows, on his scalp, and anywhere there were wrinkles on his skin. I had never heard of such a thing. The doctor prescribed a solution in which he was to be bathed three times a day. S. didn't take well to all this attention his new brother was getting from me. He became more hyperactive and refused to continue his training. In my state of panic at trying to do everything right, I did not realize at the time that this was the poor little tyke's way of coping with the new situation of losing his place in the family order. Not only was R. an intruder as far as he was concerned, but one who monopolized me. We had hired a young girl to help me in the daytime during the first three weeks of my return home with the new baby, but she did not sleep there. We could not afford full-time help, and even if we could, I would have been ashamed of not being able to cope. Every day I washed diapers in addition to having diaper service. One time I practically threw S. on the toilet seat, yelling at him that that's where he was supposed to do it. My anger must have scared him (and certainly scarred him emotionally), because after that he was trained. I still have the scene vivid in my mind. I know I could not help it. After that third birth, I cried from morning until my husband appeared after his work day. He did not have patience with my attitude. I stifled my feelings in his presence, as with everybody else. What was wrong with me? I felt like a bad person. I had fantasies of them all dying in a car accident, which made me feel even more abnormal.

At one point I got a severe pain in my abdomen. I was bent in two. I had to be hospitalized for tests because the family doctor could not figure out what was wrong with me. Again my mother refused to come and look after the children. We hired a woman who had raised nine of her own, and who, when I came back from hospital, stated she would never babysit for us again. She was exhausted. She had never seen such lively children. With disapproval in her tone of voice, she described how S. would climb up to the top of the kitchen cupboards like a monkey, as if that was bad behaviour. Three little boys full of curiosity are not easily manageable. They had to be watched every moment. No doubt they felt my nervous tension and that worsened their agitation, although R. was more placid, except for his practice of repeatedly hitting the bars of his crib with his head every night before he fell asleep. He struck with all his might. We were terrified he would hurt himself. It was another calamity I was totally unprepared for. The doctor said it would pass. I figured if we bought him a rocking horse for Christmas it might take care of what seemed to me like surplus energy. The toy was beautiful, wonderfully crafted. It worked. R. would climb on it and go at it so hard it seemed the momentum would throw him over. He loved it.

When a salesman rang the bell one day and I opened the front door, S. managed to slip past us unseen as I was talking to him. As soon as the man had left I started looking for him, but he was nowhere to be found inside or outside the house. I alerted the contractors, who organized a search in the project with their workers. Every house under construction was gone through. Nothing. I was besides myself. The police were advised of his disappearance. Speedy was overseas at the time. Several hours later, an officer phoned to say that S. had been located walking down the railroad track a couple of miles away. There were trains using that

track. I remembered that if S. stood up in his crib he could
see them pass in the distance through the window of his
bedroom. I was traumatized. It also confirmed the fact that
I could never, ever indulge in a moment of inattention as far
as looking after the children was concerned.

At the table when we were eating, Speedy had the habit
of repeatedly hitting the top of P.'s head with his index
finger when the child was misbehaving. I thought it must
hurt, but apparently it was one of the ways my husband's
own father would discipline him, and I did not have the
energy to criticize Speedy on that point. It was such a relief
for me to have him take an interest in the boys when he was
home. My mother, who happened to be visiting once and
saw him do that, took me aside and pointed out that Speedy
should not be doing that to P. Having looked after our son
after his birth, she was more attached to him than to the
other two. He was also the first grandchild. I was impressed
that she would care. It moved me to tell my husband that
if he ever did that again I would leave him. I told him to
stop picking on the child. It was then I realized Speedy had
resented the coming of our firstborn into our life, which
had considerably reduced my sexual enthusiasm. The
mention that my mother had noticed his brutality was very
convincing, and he stopped that practice.

At that point I joined a theatre group in our neighbourhood
in the hope of improving my mood. Members had to pay
$50 to the coach upon joining in order, he said, to insure
that we would attend the sessions. I related this initiative
of mine to Speedy, who incomprehensibly flew into a rage,
totally out of proportion with the sum of money involved.
Those scenes would throw me back to Father's similar,
unexplainable (in my child's mind) explosions, and I would

feel hatred for my husband because I would be overcome with dread. It was only years later I realized he was jealous of other men, or any situation he could not control where I was concerned. He need not have worried, nothing came of it. The "coach" absconded with our money.

Portrait of a Mother-in-Law

That year, Speedy's father died of cancer. We had chosen his name as R.'s second one when he was born eighteen months earlier. I thought my in-law would be pleased, but he was indifferent. He had been ill for two years, and the disease probably started in his bladder. He had seen blood in his urine, but had ignored it, too *macho* to see a doctor. He only paid attention when his legs swelled to the point of being unable to walk. The C-word would not be heard by my mother-in-law. Denial of anything unpleasant had been what carried her through life, and so the matter was never discussed with Speedy's father. She kept telling him he would get better. I suppose the doctor, realizing what a Pollyanna he was dealing with, did not have the time and the courage to set her straight.

We wondered what the shock would do to her when he died. To our great surprise, she showed no sadness at his loss. What greatly agitated her was the fact that she had to vacate the apartment she and her husband had enjoyed for free when he was superintendent of the building. They had worked for the owner for years, so she expected a pension, although it had never occurred to her before to broach the subject with the boss. Her favorite expression had been "God will provide." Since I knew damn well from the moment I was born that God never provides, and only sometimes helps those who will help themselves, I was secretly happy to see her in that predicament. After all, she had always slept very well at night while I had lied there in the throes of insomnia, worried what would happen to me for the best part of my life. She found a cheap apartment not far from where she used to live, a dump, but where she could manage financially. I found out later that Speedy sent her a cheque every month. When I did, I threw a tantrum of my own. Here I was, going to heroic lengths to be as thrifty as possible in my housekeeping, even making our milk out of powder, which the boys hated. Their allowance was pitiful compared to that of their schoolmates. I cut their hair until they rebelled. Our furniture was shabby. I felt poor and the kids felt poor, because any expense that held no direct interest for the master had to be discussed to death.

We did take them skiing in our native province during the Christmas holidays, and that was a big expense, but it was an opportunity to visit relatives on the same occasion. The stay at the resort afforded Speedy the excuse to drink plenty at dinnertime. He also enjoyed the sport and was good at it. S. was an ace, P. not bad but less agile. R. did not enjoy it, his feet being an odd shape and they were always cold, due to his boots not fitting properly. I was not a good skier. Although I pretended to enjoy the vacation, I didn't, but it was a nice change.

The reason for my indignation at my husband's largesse toward his mother is that she was a spendthrift, always blithely buying trinkets and junk when cash came her way for "gifts," mindlessly, needlessly, never wondering whether the receiver of the gift would be pleased or had any use for it. It was a selfish gesture, really, because a feeling of power always derives from buying something, as well as from giving. In the end I asked her to refrain from buying me such presents, saying it would please me more to see her spend the money on herself. I would no longer accept anything. The dinner she cooked for us on our Christmas visit would be the best gift. Speedy concurred.

Leaving Suburbia

Around that time, Speedy received another promotion, which meant we would have to move to a spot near the head office. When I learned the news I was thrilled that my husband would be given a more prestigious job with, most importantly for us, a bigger salary. At least he was fulfilling the hopes my parents and I had had for him when we married. But still my spirits remained very low. My cleaning woman admonished me: I was unhappy here in the suburbs, so why was I now complaining about moving to a new place, a new life? I got a grip on myself. The city we were moving to was nothing like the more sophisticated environment I was accustomed to. It was known as a lunch-bucket town. We made a preliminary visit to look at real estate. One of the company ladies, when I inquired about libraries, was moved to inform us that her father was a great reader and that he had read all the books ... (?) I was worried the children would lose their mother tongue.

We bought a house near the bilingual school they would attend. It was run by nuns since it belonged to the only French Catholic parish in town. It was also close to my husband's work at the company plants, which employed mostly immigrants as labourers. Therefore, our house was in a working-class district, but on a street lined with beautiful former mansions, now divided into flats previously owned by the bosses of the various steel companies. This building, still a one-unit dwelling, was from the last century. Speedy worked very hard at modernizing it, installing among other things a powder room on the first floor. It was such a contrast from our first little contemporary-style house, dreadful in its ancientness. The basement was like a dungeon, with earthen floors, a dingy toilet, with deep, stained sinks for laundry, where I found a wooden stick for poking clothes in the washing machine. I also came across a dust pan brush made of wood and real horse-hair, both antiques. I still have the laundry stick, but the brush was stolen. The boys had plenty of room to play and run around on the third floor. It even had a silent butler and stairs that divided mid-way, one part going to the back of the house, the working quarters, and the other to the front hall.

The house was very tall. It had a ledge jutting out at window-level all around the third story. One day after breakfast, Speedy having left for work and me still in my babydolls, noticed S. was not watching TV with his younger brother. I looked all over the house and spotted a window opened on the third floor. Guessing what was happening, filled with fear, I leaned through the opening, my body half out. There he was, walking along the ledge, about to disappear around a corner. I called his name softly, not wanting to startle him and see him stumble. He was enjoying himself, not listening. Controlling my terror at practically stepping into a void, I climbed out, stretched one arm, holding on to the window frame with the other one, and grabbed him, explaining we were very high up from the ground and I wouldn't want him to fall. I don't know how I did it. I spelled out that he must never, ever do that again, that it was very dangerous. I was shaking uncontrollably. I had to tell someone about having avoided a terrible accident. I immediately phoned my husband and told him what had just happened. He thought it was very funny and just laughed. He could not talk to me, he was in the middle of a meeting. He hung up. I remember as if it was yesterday how rage and loneliness engulfed me simultaneously.

My fears about my children losing the language were justified. They soon realized the other kids spoke English in school even at recreation time, and since their father used it as well, it became their language of choice. I always spoke and answered them in French, to the great puzzlement of their little friends who, many of them, had no idea what it was, which I think embarrassed the boys, but I persisted. I did not insist they use it themselves, fearing they would not talk to me. After all, I was not running a language school. The greatest problem as far as school was concerned was that the Catholic religion was still dominant and domineering outside my native province, where we had succeeded in shaking its yoke. The nuns and the parish priest, upon hearing my better educated way of speaking than what they were accustomed to from the rest of the flock, and my self-assurance compared to that of a more subservient community, did not like me. They ignored me when I tried to engage in conversation. That was not good for our boys, who asked too many questions in class and appeared more knowledgeable than their teachers.

When we moved, we brought our skis, leaving them on the back porch, which provoked the question from our neighbours: What are you going to do here with those? At the time, the city hardly ever got any snow in the winter, but the next year it came in such abundance that a little

T-lift was installed on the golf course to take advantage of the escarpment. This little hill was frequented with great enthusiasm by the locals, making them feel worldly at tackling such an international sport. I went a couple of times at night myself to relieve the tediousness of my days in a city which showed no foreign films, and where the library, as I was advised, only carried books which were "in demand by the people." It was pointed out as I specified I was looking for Virginia Woolf's diaries that this library was "an institution for the general public."

Not long after we arrived, Speedy invited some of his superiors for cocktails at our house. They were all sitting in the living room, and I was in the kitchen preparing hors d'oeuvres to serve them. His former boss inquired of my husband how I was. Speedy replied, "She's fine, all she needs is a good kick in the ass," as I was entering the room with the tray. I saw the former's face flush in anger. He got up and said, "If you ever talk like that about your wife again, I'll hit you." What a gentleman! And what a prick Speedy revealed himself to be in front of everyone. Again, he was playing the tough guy. It was not funny, but I pretended to take it as a joke, to save embarrassment

I never got used to the town, although we were engulfed in a social whirl which I had never known before. Through one of Speedy's colleagues (who knew a lot of people at the university), we joined a circle of friends, none of them native to the area, from all parts of the world, who had known the war, who were cultured and interesting. They had what I had always sought in relationships. We entertained a lot, and my cooking was praised. We knew about good wines. Our presence was sought. Speedy was a good talker, keeping conversations lively, his conservative opinions clashing with those of our liberal-minded friends, and he charmed the ladies with his good looks, seductive compliments, and pipe. Although my secret angst remained, I was sure this (novel for me) popularity would cure it.

A Stricken Child

When R. was six years old, he contracted acute osteomyelitis, an infection of the bone through bacteria. I noticed it as I was giving him a bath. One of his shoulder blades was sticking out a bit more than the other. He was given antibiotics immediately and hospitalized for three weeks. It was early September and he was about to enter Grade 1. I went to the school and asked the teacher to lend me the books she would be using to start. I took them to the hospital on my visits and went over the reading material he would have been learning in class. He loved it and made good progress. When he was cured and came home, he appeared to be back to his normal self. It was now time for him to go to school like other children his age. He did not take to it; being taught in a class of over twenty pupils is quite different from learning one on one. Starting school is hard enough in normal circumstances. I was torn. I did not realize he could have been suffering from psychological trauma, being my usual distraught self. Had I felt stable as I do today, I would have kept him at home for a little while longer. I feel bad about it still.

A New Neighbourhood

When P. reached Grade 8 (which was not offered at the bilingual school), and our car (which we had to park on the street) was hit by an unknown driver on our narrow boulevard, I had also reached a point where I couldn't stand the nuns' attitude toward us and the lamentable quality of teaching in what was an inner-city school, where my progeny had nothing in common with the other kids, who spoke neither language properly. We moved to a house in an upscale neighbourhood across the street from the university. Our new address impressed our friends, but our furniture certainly did not match our improved abode. My husband, who had been raised in shabby surroundings, did not see the necessity of spending any more money on a respectable interior. What mattered most to him was his work. Insisting would have meant endless arguments which I was not prepared to undertake. I was happy enough, nay, grateful, with our new environment, but the contrast bothered me. I resented it. I was afraid people would think we were living above our means, which was contemptible in those days. I did not earn any money, and I had little say in the matter, never using sex as leverage. Father, who had visited before we purchased the place, provided an interest-free loan to help us finance the mortgage. He had inspected the dwelling and was more than satisfied with the quality of the materials in the forty-year-old building and the location of the house. He was very proud of the improvement in our status.

The children started going to the local high school, which enjoyed high academic standards, given the community was part Jewish, part upscale WASPs, with the university nearby, and with a smattering of working-class families. Our neighbours on both sides and in our immediate vicinity were professors. The second family to buy the house on our right was made up of a teaching psychiatrist from down under whose wife had been a psychiatrist nurse, and both were more or less bonkers. When she found a shoe on the curb in front of her house, she insisted to me that someone had been kidnapped the night before, and nagged me endlessly about doing something about it, saying that we should call the police. She was bigger than her husband and dominated him entirely. When she became aware of the way our Siberian Husky attracted attention because of his beauty and pedigree, they acquired a gorgeous young Irish setter which ran around like crazy. It was unmanageable, as that breed is wont to be, but so lovable that the husband fell in love with the creature, at which point she made him get rid of it. When we purchased our Jaguar XKE, she made him buy a Mercedes convertible, the first such model. He also had to purchase a hot pink Volkswagen Beetle, so she "could keep track of him in town." She had insinuated that she suspected Speedy and her spouse were having an affair.

At five o'clock one morning, our doorbell rang insistently. When I opened it, I was confronted with the spectacle of my psychiatrist neighbour covered in blood. "She has beaten me up," he moaned. "Help me." It upset me. I was aware that I was being asked to partake of their sadomasochistic game, an activity which was not that much in vogue in those days. I called Speedy, not knowing what to do with the doctor. He walked him back home and reasoned with the wife with a straight face. I knew he thought the whole incident was a big joke. We both felt nothing but contempt for the antics of the couple, but had not suspected they were that far gone in their kinkiness. He called her "a dirty flash." They moved out of town back to where she came from shortly after that incident to "start anew." I heard later from someone close to the faculty that they were a swinging couple, and that she was into Satanism. They might have been asked to leave; I was not the only one who found them strange. Apparently they had a bad reputation in the ivory tower.

Years later, when we weren't living there anymore, Speedy asked me to read an article he had just perused in a weekend magazine. "Anything you recognize in that piece?" he asked. Upon paying more attention, the name of my former female neighbour jumped at me. It was an unusual name I had never heard before or since. No doubt now about whom this was referring to. It was the story of the disappearance of a university professor's wife and the subsequent discovery overseas of her remains in a green garbage bag. The wife had accompanied her professor husband to a conference in a European country and had suddenly vanished from the scene. During the police investigation that followed, it was discovered that my ex-neighbour was a student of the professor, subsequently becoming his mistress, and secretly joining him at the conference. According to the article, the police were never able to establish beyond a reasonable doubt who perpetrated the crime, and the professor got off scot-free. They did not know his mistress as well as I did. At the time, she was still married to her psychiatrist husband. Case closed, I suppose. When they lived next to us, they first had a little girl, and then a little boy was born. After he was able to walk, the girl would lure him to the side of their house which had no windows – I could view this from mine – and torture him.

Before moving away, they had sold their house to a specialist in cardiology who was famous for his research on cholesterol. His near and dear took this notion very seriously: no beef, no eggs, no butter, absolutely no animal fat, and you would never, never have a heart attack. They believed that implicitly. I admired such faith, but thought it was utter nonsense. I never went for it. They had three sons exactly the same age as ours. I wished they would be friends. It was not possible. They were getting better allowances than we gave our kids. They were also Jewish Orthodox and did not mix with Gentiles. The mother was someone important in the women's world of the temple. She appeared miffed when we gave a party which turned out to be particularly rambunctious – one of our guests had disappeared when his wife was ready to go home, and was found the next day sleeping it off in a car in one of the university's parking lots. I apologized for the noise our guests made when taking leave in the wee hours, and realized she would have liked to be invited. Since they had never made any social gesture toward us, I had not thought they were interested. Nevertheless, they did offer sympathy when our youngest went on his rampage, saying they understood, that their own kids had gotten in trouble with the law a couple of times over drugs. Mighty nice of them. They were also lucky —they won the jackpot in the lottery twice.

On the other side of our house there lived first a chemistry professor and family, British, who went back to their country every summer and whose dream was to move back to England. They were also Jewish but non- practicing, and they were already part of our social circle. I was fond of the wife, although I deplored her habit of handing her baby girls lollipops the minute they started crying, even if it did have the desired effect of shutting them up. By the time their father was offered a position in a famous university in Britain, they were obese little girls, as was their mother.

Him I had never liked. He always seemed to be in a bad mood. "He's very low today," she would invariably offer to explain his rudeness. Maybe he sensed that I found him physically repugnant. For some reason his face reminded me of a pig, although the actual animal does not have that effect on me. I always wondered how she could bring herself to have sex with him, but then the prestige of being married to a university professor made everything all right; such is the female imperative. Pretend. Although in those days of vocal feminism, it was at last recognized that a woman had a right to lust and to get something physical herself out of lying down with a man. A lot of them still did not acknowledge their needs. Nowadays some teenage girls blithely service the boys in exchange for popularity. Little has changed.

When they left for England, those neighbours sold their house to another professor. He was part of a young couple, just married, WASPs this time, very prim and proper, very straight. The wife, a goodie-goodie type, was in a continuous blissful state, as attested by the beatific smile which almost never left her face, induced, I think, by the fact that they owned this glorious Tudor-style house with large grounds in our upscale neighborhood right across the street from the university where she worked as a lab technician. Her felicity could not have come from his personality; he was a creep, always leering at me. When I attended to the thirty rose bushes which lined our long driveway on Sundays (in my bathing suit if it was a hot summer day), he would manage to find something to do on that side of their house and stare at me. He was the kind of man who, when our youngest was arrested and friends came to our house to commiserate and offer support, leaned against his car outside in his driveway, taking in the show with a triumphant smile on his face. I never knew what he had against us. He probably did not approve of our sons' rock band in the basement, or my attending university. Many years later, after we had moved, I ran into them at the grocery store I still occasionally frequented in that neighbourhood. The whole family, father, mother, daughter, and son, was there, not speaking to each other and looking grim, the teenagers especially, with that hostile look on their faces. Life had done its work. I was pleased.

Every summer they would take off for the West, where they hailed from, for a month, and rent their house. One particular couple of tenants from Australia sticks in my memory. The owner had a vegetable garden, the proceeds of which I had of course never seen, but the male tenant took to coming over and offering me huge zucchinis from their crop. I would thank him profusely, wondering whether I should be insulted. I did not know how Speedy would take this generosity toward his wife, but the message was so clear, and funny, that he was just as amused as I was, as were other people I reported this to.

Teenagers

When the children were still with us, we used to go back up North every Christmas holiday, combining visits to family and skiing. We all enjoyed it, especially the dog who, being a Siberian Husky, just loved the snow. We enjoyed the trips until the boys were well into their teens and started smoking pot. After that, everything became a bore for them. I was never a good skier. Having started when I was very young, I was unable of getting rid of bad habits I had acquired when the sport consisted mainly of going straight down a hill and making turns with your waist instead of using the knees, as is now the technique. I was always cold, but I gamely partook, stiff with the fear of falling, crashing regularly, devoid of control, ending up black and blue, but persisting in my longing to do things together as a family. Getting on or off the ski lift also terrified me. I fell down a couple of times. The machine had to be stopped. It was very embarrassing. One day, ten years later, as I stood at the top of the mountain about to take my run down, I lost it, admitted this was not for me, never had been, for lack of form. Courage I had had. No more. I never skied downhill again. Cross-country became my winter sport while Speedy continued downhill. It was lonely out there in the woods, and I really never quite enjoyed it until I left him and became more relaxed. S. was extraordinarily good at the sport, being so agile and fearless, climber that he was.

We took the boys to Expo '67 and to the Olympic Games. I have pictures, but I don't remember those being happy occasions. It was forced entertainment. I wanted to do things to make them happy, but my always being on edge over Speedy's drinking the moment he had an idle moment and my lack of sleep had to affect them. We camped in a tent trailer Speedy had built, and which he was rightly very proud of.

The only thing that kept me going in those days was the idea of grandchildren. No doubt due to the tense atmosphere in our home (the absentee father and the always morose mother), combined with the fact that they had not found their niche in the new school, our two younger sons started smoking cannabis and hashish. P., having started in that institution one year before they did, had found a group of like nerds and was quite comfortable with them. He also made friends with the son of a French-speaking professor and would spend most of his evenings at their house. I suspect they were into magic mushrooms, but doping had not yet become a plague. Parents were not aware of it. The professor was an inveterate alcoholic with no wife, living with a female graduate student. Nevertheless, years later, during one of those periods when I was attempting to rid myself of Speedy and we were separated, I ran into the professor at one of the French community's meetings. He invited me to be his date at some university affair. I gladly accepted – he was very handsome in spite of being a lush, and I was vulnerable and confused. Not having heard from him (I should have known better), I phoned his house to confirm. His student answered: No, he had not mentioned anything about that. She was the one going with him. This female student managed to put up with him for years and finally got him to marry her. Last I heard he had sobered up. She had hung on to him and had won.

By the time I was doing my Master's, pot was all the rage amongst high school and university students. One fellow in my French literature class was a maverick who had come from the mathematics department and who befriended me, most likely because I was so different from our nubile cohorts. We had philosophical discussions. One day during my doctoral studies in the big city, I ran into him on the street, and he was so stoned I could not get a coherent sentence out of him. I asked him what he was doing now, what field he was in. He recognized me and seemed embarrassed, even in his high state, conscious of his lamentable condition. He was a mess, straggly hair, eyes so red, stumbling. I thought he was doomed. Then, about fifteen years later, as I was taking an evening walk in the last neighbourhood where I lived in that city, on a pretty street I had never explored before, I recognized him coming out of a pleasant middle-class bungalow and stopped him. He did not seem to recall who I was at first. He explained he was now a medical doctor on his way to the famous health center in our town. He was married, it seemed, with a family, and that bungalow was his house. I was flabbergasted. He had one strange eye which made him look sinister, and you never knew if he was with you or laughing at you.

During P.'s last year in high school I started worrying about a strange habit of his which I had mentioned to every family doctor we had ever had without getting anywhere, because you had to witness the occurrence several times to grasp that something was not quite right. I was invariably told that it would pass. Whenever P. got excited about something, his hands would start fluttering along his sides and he would fall into some kind of a trance. I would have to loudly utter his name for him to snap out of it. It looked like he was not aware of those uncontrolled moments. I was afraid that when he attended university his fellow students would make fun of him. I broached the subject with the doctor who was head of our family unit at the health center. Since it was something which was difficult to describe and he did not seem to understand what I was talking about, I suggested that perhaps P. suffered from *petit mal*, a form of epilepsy not as dramatic as the convulsive one. Perhaps I sounded impatient with the physician; he took umbrage at my knowledge and stated I had no business telling him how to do his job. Two days later we received a letter from him advising me that he refused to treat our family anymore because he and I were not compatible, that I had broken the bond of trust essential to a doctor/patient relationship. I was stunned, dismayed, and profoundly disturbed, not knowing what to do.

At that time I was giving private French language lessons to a specialist high up in the hospital's administration. In my state of distress I could not help relating the incident to him. He became highly indignant and stated that if one of his children was sick, he would have done exactly the same. He said he would take care of the whole situation, and not to worry. He assigned us a new family doctor and arranged for my husband to take the boy to the Johns Hopkins Institute for diagnosis. Speedy drove P. to that institution in Maryland, where a series of tests were performed on our son, one of which featured an epidural which left him semi-unconscious for several days. The tests were inconclusive. The specialist pronounced that the condition was "probably" a form of epilepsy and prescribed medication to that effect. Unfortunately, the cure was worse than the disease. P. became a zombie, unable to study, looking haggard, livid, hardly able to speak, and so pitiful it was breaking my heart. After six months of that regime I could not take it anymore, and I advised our family doctor in no uncertain terms that as far as I was concerned, the treatment was an aberration, that it was ruining our son's life as well as his future, and that he was better off going back to his previous ineffable habit. The medical man had to agree with my reasoning and we gradually decreased the dosage of P.'s medication until he returned to his normal self. He did suffer terrible pranks played on him at university, and I felt so sorry for him. He was a nice guy and very generous, having succeeded very well in his profession, enjoying his own version of the revenge of the nerds. I can't help but think, though: why did my motherhood involve so many crosses to bear? One thing after another.

I could smell the pot on my kids' clothes, which were often not the ones they had started with in the morning. When I confronted them, they would deny it. As for their father, if he thought it was serious, he had more important things to deal with. He wouldn't have a sit-down talk with them. Contrary to their older brother, they had fallen in with a bad crowd. I sensed they felt disconnected. Having to move from classroom to classroom, with different teachers and students for each subject, contrary to elementary school, does not help. Money started disappearing from my wallet. One day I found a new jacket with the price tag still attached in R.'s closet. He admitted taking it from a store. "What on earth for?" I cried. To give it to a friend at school, he said. I assumed it was to ingratiate himself with the said friend, more likely in exchange for pot, I now realize. Together, we brought the garment back to the store owner with apologies from, and embarrassment for, us both. Nowadays I wonder if they didn't also ditch the very healthy lunches I prepared every morning for them to take to school in favor of the junk food sold in the cafeteria. They might have felt dorky eating carrots instead of fries. Hence the need for a bigger allowance.

In order to counter bad peer influence and the use of drugs, I offered up our basement as a venue for rock band practice. This way I would know where my children were. S. played the guitar and R. was the "singer." For months they blasted off down there. The neighbours on whose side there were windows were none too pleased. However heroic my efforts were to ingratiate my teenagers in that way, the plan backfired and did not prevent disaster. We were robbed twice during that period. The kids did not always lock the basement door when they left, and the other members of the band, not being of the same fortunate background as our boys, were in fact hostile to our lifestyle – I felt it in the sneering way they addressed me – which made us vulnerable to that kind of intrusion.

They were just using our sons for a place to play. S. was kicked out of the band as soon as they found another local to practice. It was a huge blow to him, from which I'm not sure he recovered for a long time. He joined another group whose music was too avant-garde for the times and failed to attract attention. I deeply felt for S. He nevertheless attended the local university for a couple of years after that. After what happened with his younger brother, his substance abuse seemed to disappear. R. did not stay with the band that long. It would seem that he had always felt like an outsider, even in company of his two older brothers, in the sense that "three is a crowd." He had pestered the group to join them, thus being designated the singer, a feature which they lacked, already having enough instrumentalists.

The Rampage

R. has never wanted to discuss with us or a psychiatrist the reason why he and three other teenagers who were in one of his classes at school, not even close friends, went on a rampage, vandalizing five houses in our district. In all five, the owners were away. The boys started drinking in the conservation area bordering our neighbourhood, and then went looking for more booze, breaking and entering, damaging the premises as they did so. Apparently drugs were not involved. Had they consumed hash or pot, the kids wouldn't have become violent, trying to out-do each other in daring feats. The reaction in town was vicious. Gate-crashing at parties when parents were away had not been invented yet, and this event was, in our midst, the first occurrence of youth wantonness. It was as if an atomic bomb in all it unexpectedness and amplitude had been dropped on our population. My work in the courts confirmed later that damage to property is much more abhorrent to our society than physical violence. The boys were arrested the next day and remanded, as they should be, but this was an experience I had absolutely never in my life envisaged.

The morning before, a couple of policemen had banged on our door and looked around for evidence. I was still unaware of what had taken place, and had a towel wrapped around my head after washing my hair. They offered no explanation as to why they were there. One of them savagely kicked the boots and overshoes in the entrance closet. He seized a pair of yellow work ones, Kodiacs, that, as he put it, the bastard must have been wearing when he committed his crime. I did not know what the policeman was talking about. R. had come home the evening before, his surly self as usual (he had a part-time job at McDonald's), had not said anything, and supposedly left for school in the morning. Speedy was away on business at the time. There had been no previous hint of this spectacularly rebellious gesture which would change R.'s life forever. Things had appeared normal in our dysfunctional family.

For the last five years I had been driving thirty-five miles three times a week to work as a graduate teaching assistant to indifferent students, writing my thesis, barely sustained by the hope that someday I would become a professor and get out of my marriage. Running a household and studying for my Ph.D. was a harrowing combination, but not enough of an escape to keep me unaware that the boys were unhappy. I felt helpless where they were concerned. Nothing I said ever seemed to register with them, perhaps because they were witness to the fact that their father was forever contradicting me, intimating that I was a nag. It seemed to me that I was merely trying to instill in them the values I had been brought up with. P. was away at university by then. The odd thing is that two of the other teens, brothers, who participated in the rampage, came from what appeared to me to be a loving environment. We socialized with the parents. The mother gave piano lessons at home. The father was a professor at the university, an alcoholic, but whose wife didn't mind his drinking. I envied and admired her for that, having never been able to accept that weakness in a man, probably because of what I had endured with Father. Any kind of substance abuse will send me into a frenzy. I watched Speedy's imbibing like a hawk, always on the alert, which made for much tension in my life, but it certainly kept him sober for functioning and performing above average at his work, for achieving his potential. They can all thank me for that, but what a toll it took on my nerves. Without me harping about it, he would have drunk continually, as he did when he was idle on holidays or traveling on business.

This traumatic event provided much welcome fodder for the town's newspaper, which milked the story for all it was worth. I was devastated, not so much by the fact that I received hate phone calls — some stating that if I didn't try to be something other than a housewife this would not have happened — and at least one death threat, but by the fact it confirmed the abysmal emotional misery my children had in common with me, which added to my distress. Having always been able to put myself in other peoples' places, I visualized what the victims must have felt when they returned and found their homes invaded and trashed. I remembered how, after the first robbery, every time I came in the door upon returning from a trip out of town I was terrified I would find the place ransacked, a feeling of having been violated, which lasted until we moved to another part of the city. Ironically, it never happened there, although the house itself was more contemporary and filled with luxury items. Our former residence didn't contain much worth taking (I was not employed yet, had no money to decorate nicely, and Speedy was not forthcoming with funds for that purpose, since it was not important to him) except for the silver, which we had inherited from both sides of the family, and which indeed was lifted to the single last piece. The first set of thieves, who entered by breaking down the back door with the axe lying around on the back porch, took it all. The robbers overlooked a beautiful genuine Wedgewood cookie jar featuring a silver handle and ball feet supporting a blue ceramic container, where cavorted in relief white figures of antiquity. Obviously the thieves had no idea of its worth. I was thrilled to find it intact. My ex-husband has it now, since it came from his family.

Being totally inexperienced in the judicial world, we went to a lawyer friend of ours for our son's defense in the bail hearing. He was extremely reluctant to take the case, criminal law not being his specialty, and not being a courtroom lawyer. He probably suggested someone more qualified to do the job, but we were so ignorant of such matters, so troubled and so in need of a sympathetic environment, that we insisted on his services. Out of pity for us he finally accepted, no doubt warning us that he was not up to it. But we just didn't understand. For us, one advocate was as good as another, not aware that there are specialties in law just as in medicine. Only years later, when ironically I was appointed to a position in the judicial system, did I realize how stupid we had been.

The bail hearing took place. Because none of the kids had a criminal record, they were released on a surety pledged by us, and with very strict conditions: R. was a virtual prisoner in our house, not being allowed to go out and, among other things, was ordered to abstain from alcoholic beverages. He didn't take well at all to losing his freedom. From surly teenager that he was before, he became very hostile, with no remorse whatsoever. No comforting or conciliatory effort on my part seemed to reach him. We were stuck together in the house whenever I was not at the university or doing errands. The tension was palpable. One time he left the house without me, contrary to the court's order, was away for hours, and came back quite drunk. I should have reported it to the police, but of course I didn't. I'm not sure I was fully aware at the time I was supposed to do so, that bail conditions were binding. I was still in a state of shock. I certainly did not want the boy to think I was against him. Speedy was out of town most of the time and even when he was home, the fact that he went to work every day meant that he did not have to face the situation, hour after hour. He was glad to get away, to forget about it, to lose himself in his work. He never mentioned his colleagues' reaction to the event. In a way, I can understand his trying to forget about the whole thing, but it made the burden all mine. Perhaps his long ago association with petty criminals and the street life of his youth made him more impervious to this brush with the law I suddenly found myself immersed in.

Another irony: the policeman who barged into our house on that day appeared before me in criminal court twenty years later, twice, for his own bail hearings regarding two different incidents of violence. I recognized him, although I never knew his name, and prayed he did not recognize me and remind the public of my son's crime. Defendants who were acquainted with me outside the courtroom for some reason or other, or because of repeat appearances, invariably hailed me from the dock, sometimes expansively, outbursts which of course I ignored, but it would have been pretty tricky for me in this case. He didn't recognize me. I would not have been fired for something that someone in my family had done, but certainly now that I think of it, it would have put me in a conflict of interest, not to mention the shame that would have engulfed me all over again. In fact, from the first day I started officiating in the courts on a regular basis, I lived in dread that someone would link my son's surname to mine.

After a few years I realized that since, by its very nature, the judicial environment consists of dealing with an unending succession of criminal matters, the chance of R.'s delinquent activities resurfacing in any law-connected individual's memory were minimal. As soon as a matter is dealt with, it is filed away to make room for the new ones, given the backload, and promptly forgotten. There is no time for lingering, especially with all the guilty pleas which, necessarily, intentionally, make the machine go even faster, in order to deal with all the cases. Who can, who wants to remember what was dealt with last month, never mind twenty years ago? In any case, something else more traumatizing happened some thirteen years later in the exercise of my judicial functions which would brutally eclipse that first brush with the law through my boy's misconduct.

Some Lawyers

The brother of that wayward policeman who had long ago arrested my son was an assistant crown-attorney in our region, which made the matter of the accused policeman very sensitive and juicy, because this brother was consistently being reprimanded for leering lecherously at his female colleagues, be they other prosecutors or defense attorneys or even defendants. The reason he kept his job, as did one other crown-attorney who consorted with a prostitute, is that the system is desperately short of prosecutors. To be fair, defense lawyers were also forgiven, as was the coke-head who beat his female companion to a pulp in a hotel room, as was the one who was found smuggling dope to prisoners at the local detention center. Another lawyer was involved in a sordid trial *à la* Michael Johnson, and who, as I expected after reading about his accusers, was acquitted: the arguments as formulated by his defense counsel would create a reasonable doubt in the minds of the jury. In this case, the "victims" were male teenagers who accused the attorney (representing them under Legal Aid) of forcing them to perform oral sex on him whenever they were in his office. This came as a shock to his wife who, in extreme denial, outrage, and loyalty, protested, proclaimed and swore to his heterosexuality. After all, they had children together. Equally shocked was his partner in the law firm they co-owned together. It was, of course, a crime of abuse of authority, since the accused claimed the participants in the *fellatio* sessions were consenting in gratifying him with blow jobs. I believe his argument in persuading them to service him was that he could protect them from the police. At this time, the firm also let go on some pretext or other of one of their young lawyers who happened to be openly homosexual. Many people in the system already knew the accused was gay. I did, for a long time. A young crown-attorney friend of mine, also gay, had once confided in me that the accused was known to cruise the strip male prostitutes frequented, which to his surprise I did not even know existed in our town.

Eventually, after a few years, this homosexual lawyer who had restricted his extra-marital activities since he had been acquitted at his trial (his defense to the effect that his so-called victims were ruffians, prostitutes, and drug addicts, and therefore not credible, was endorsed by the jury) resumed his same-sex activities. I saw him engage in flirtation with another gay member at our local Y. It was quite a ballet of seduction, with the other guy batting eyelashes and all, and our lawyer friend ending up waiting for his sex partner in the lobby. His wife finally resigned herself to his sexual orientation and agreed to a divorce. I wonder what they told the kids.

The profession, like any other, takes care of its own. With scandals like that popping up periodically but regularly, who can remember them all? The cop in question was being prosecuted twenty years after he had arrested our son and his accomplices. This policeman was now addled by his long abuse of alcohol, and most likely other substances, and was incoherent in court. The first time he was released by another magistrate to the custody of his parents on a recognizance and a surety, he was perfectly aware he was committing himself to abide by the conditions of his bail or his parents would have to pay the amount they pledged in exchange for his release. He disobeyed the court orders several times, each time hauled back for a new bail hearing, until out of pity for his folks as much as for his being repeatedly oblivious to his obligations — he certainly had been treated with more indulgence than a civilian — he was remanded until his trial. He must have pled guilty in exchange for a very short sentence. Jail wouldn't be kind to an ex-cop.

The Criminal

Although our son and his partners in crime pled not guilty, they were of course found so, and sentenced to six months in jail. I would visit him once a week, alternating with Speedy. He, of course, was not as flexible with regards to visiting hours. Those were very difficult moments. The way the room was set up it made it practically impossible to have a conversation: there was an open slot at the bottom of the window of individual booths, where both the visitor and the prisoner had to bend down in order to communicate in an impossibly uncomfortable position. It was very undignified, with everybody's posteriors sticking out. At the time, it struck me as being totally absurd that an arrangement meant for conversation could be so badly designed with total disregard for its users. In those days, still being unacquainted with the correctional services, I was not aware that humane considerations did not at all enter into the equation. On those visits R. was even more sullen than ever. If he was happy to see me, it didn't show. He complained endlessly, as if he hadn't landed himself where he was. Because he was defiant with the guards and totally uncooperative, a troublemaker, he had to serve almost his whole six months instead of being released in a much shorter time. I know his accomplices fared better than he did. He thought they were kiss-ass with the screws. I tried to explain to him that things would be easier for him if he behaved nicely, even if in my mind I thought the guards were probably sadistic buggers.

The jail was supposed to provide schooling, but they were short of books and the teacher only attended once a week. At least that's what R. reported to me. Whether he was making the effort or not, I don't know. Prison is not like a hospital where you can discuss the welfare of the patient with the doctors and nurses. In a detention center, the authorities don't give a shit, especially if the inmate comes from a privileged background. It seems rehabilitation is a concern only in penitentiaries. It was a jolt to me every time I had to ring the bell to get buzzed in, in order to be admitted on the premises for a visit. What a lesson in humility!

When he was released, his old school would not take R. back. We found one in another part of town which reluctantly accepted him. He had lost one year. He was treated like a pariah in the new one, which did not help matters. The principal told us he had fallen in with a bad bunch, was skipping school again. No wonder: the good guys would not have anything to do with him. He was a jailbird. After a while he refused to go back. He was by now seventeen and had not completed Grade 10.

The judge at the bail hearing had ordered family therapy, but no psychiatrist in town wanted to take us on, claiming they did not have the expertise to deal with our case. In reality, they were disgusted with us. They had never before encountered youths of their own social class who had engaged in criminal activities. The term "dysfunctional" had not entered their professional jargon yet. Runaway, rebellious, or dope-consuming teens had not become an entrenched social phenomenon.

My husband and I were all for therapy. We finally found a doctor who agreed to see us, but he also made it very clear that he was doing us a big favour, showing an obvious distaste for getting involved with the likes of us. I would soon realize why. In the meantime, Speedy and I were ever so relieved and full of hope in having found treatment for what ailed us. Our youngest sons would get back on the right track. There was a light at the end of the tunnel. We attended a few sessions, which did not go very well, because R. scorned the whole process. He did not take to the shrink, who, I felt, without mentioning it, was judgmental. On trial day this doctor, who was not a witness, showed up in court; I was gratified that he cared enough to forego his office hours until I saw his wife sitting there beside him. So, they viewed this event that was torture for us parents of the accused as a show. And then I noticed the woman had her hair wrapped in a kerchief: Orthodox Jews. I was crestfallen. How could this man ever empathize with a family where the wife is studying for a Ph.D. while his own was by religious dictate considered impure when menstruating, separated from the male congregation in the synagogue, never allowed to question her status or fate? I confronted him with those facts at the next session and voiced serious doubts about his ability to understand the dynamics of our family, where I was striving for equality. Thus ended the therapy.

His father gave R. an ultimatum which I supported: Either attend school or find a job, otherwise you can't live here anymore. Speedy thought this tactic would work, but I did not have such confidence. R. seemed to hate us so, but I was willing to try anything to find a resolution. R. chose to leave. He did so with glee. He was showing us he didn't need us, that it would be fantastic being free of all authority.

Since birth, R. had suffered from psoriasis, but refused all treatments that were available at the time, such as my washing his hair with a special solution. Even years later, when for a while I regained contact with him, he wouldn't pay any attention when I apprised him of the treatments that were now available for his condition, although he was ashamed of it and was convinced no girl would ever look at him. He was so handsome, as I kept telling him. A year later, when more and more teens of "respectable" backgrounds were playing hooky, an alternative school was founded which administered "tough love," a method which seemed to work. It was too late for our son, with whom we had lost touch. At one point, he was living in a friend's house whose parents had died. I bought them groceries once after running into R. on the street. He was not so cocky anymore. He was very scruffy and playing the martyr, but showing no sign of being willing to compromise. Then when that arrangement no longer worked, he lived on the street.

Since his arrest, I had been living in an acute state of anxiety, compounded now by my worry of what was going to happen to him. The only respite was my studies, although the economy was now entering a recession and the universities tightened their hiring. What had looked like a cinch when I started my B.A. (becoming a professor after completing my Ph.D.) had become doubtful, but after ten years of successful studies and overcoming obstacles, I could not give it up. To the sadness of losing a son, which I considered a personal failure, was added the dismaying inkling of the futility in pursuing my dream.

PART THREE

A Second Career

Academe

I've always felt extremely fortunate to have experienced university life. It had been such a heartbreaker when in my late teens I had been denied that privilege. This aspiration materialized in my late thirties only because I was giving French conversation lessons to a friend of ours who was a sociology professor at the campus located across the street from our house. We had agreed to meet at the Faculty Club once a week and speak French, which he sort of knew since he originated from Montreal. One day he asked why I didn't go back to school and get a university degree. I had mentioned to him how much I regretted not having been allowed to pursue advanced studies. I was not aware such an endeavour was a possibility. I don't know if he really meant this advice, but I took it seriously. I discussed it with my husband, who seemed amenable to the idea, for which

I was grateful. I did not realize at the time, although I was aware of the huge chip on his shoulder about not having a degree, especially since the people we frequented socially were almost all university professors with Ph.D.s, that even though he seemed to approve of my project there would be hell to pay if I engaged in an activity which would confer upon me something he didn't have, such as a university diploma. He may have thought when I mentioned my desire to go back to school I would not persist beyond a B.A., if it even went that far.

I was much more worried about passing the tests in order to be admitted than in pondering the consequences of my bettering myself. I was sure I would fail anyway, since the math part was bound to be way beyond anything I had learned in school at the end of the forties in a girls-only institution. I had hated the elementary algebra the nuns taught us. Anything to do with numbers was the bane of my life, although I had not done too badly in physics and geometry. To this day I have absolutely no memory for digits. And indeed I was unable to answer the questions in the math section of the admission test, but having done exceptionally well in every other subject, as a "mature student," I was deemed acceptable. Academic institutions always have a great need for funds. I was overjoyed.

Attending university was something I had longed for all those years, but I had butterflies in my stomach on registration day. I was almost paralyzed by the thought of my temerity in undertaking such a life change. It was a notion unheard of. No other woman with children as far as I knew had yet attempted it. My three boys were in school full day by that time, and all I had to do was cross the street to attend my various classes. But panic overtook me when the professor in History 101 went through the list of books we had to read (and therefore buy) for that course. It struck me as very expensive, as well as leaving no time to write the essays also required of us. And that was just one course. Innocent me, I did not know that professors in the same field were in the habit of recommending each other's works, a practice which boosted the number of sales of their respective publications and therefore advancement. I had never heard the phrase "publish or perish." I was entering a whole new world full of wonders, such as acquiring knowledge, and of perils, such as how I would be perceived by faculty and students, being the first wife and mother taking daytime courses in a regular honours programme (at least in that provincial university).

My first year toward getting a B.A. was 1967, before students had started wearing jeans. Being stoned on pot for days was unheard of, the sexual revolution had not taken place, and feminism was in its infancy. I was the first woman in that factory town to attempt combining family, housework, and full-time post-secondary studies toward a degree. It was extremely difficult. It was heroic. Especially because I didn't sleep. Looking back on it, I don't know how I did it. It was insane, but it was my chance to satisfy my enduring intellectual curiosity. I had been a truly desperate housewife. I was convinced this endeavour would abate the beast gnawing inside me, and bring me if not happiness at least the serenity marriage had failed to provide. As the years passed and I proceeded to acquire one degree after another, the project formed in my mind to carry this quest to its logical and legitimate end and become a university professor myself. As far as I was concerned, based on observation, they enjoyed the ideal life: teaching six months a year with time off for Christmas holidays and student reading week, free time for research for three months during the summer, and after their first year of teaching a course, no subsequent preparation on the subject seemed to be expected (at the time). All through my seventeen years as a student in the humanities, the classes were a reasonable size, and the pressure was not on as it is now to pass students at all costs, at the risk of being sued if they were failed. On the other hand, the concept of sexual harassment did not exist yet.

My dwelling in the ivory tower certainly was an eye-opener. So far I had led a somewhat sheltered life, having passed from the authority of my parents and the nuns to that of a husband with only a short interlude of four years working in an office. There, I had been humbled, it's true, but I attributed that to the fact that I couldn't type and was not amongst my peers.

Like a lot of people ignorant of that environment, I was under the impression that academe was a matrix for knowledge as well as a bastion of virtue. I discovered at my own emotional expense what a jungle it was out there among the scholars. When I confronted a professor with the fact that she had given me a B on an essay, the same mark which a regular student (as opposed to myself, as a mature student) had achieved, whose paper I had read to see if it was as good as mine, and which I found to be incoherent, my own work being tightly and logically structured according to the way I had been taught in my youth, I protested to her that her marking was unfair. How naïve and foolish of me! Her reply was that I should know by now, at my age, that life is indeed unfair, that she was rewarding not the end results but said student's efforts and "creativity." Besides, he was "so cute."

I was dumbfounded. Excellence, which I had always thought was the criterion, didn't count. Obviously, my particular circumstances of getting a degree while carrying on with my other duties did not weigh at all when it came to efforts being deployed to produce the required scholastic work. Very disheartening. I expected some recognition of my struggle, and success in spite of my special status. That recognition never came, the attitude from faculty was resentment, and from the students, bafflement. A similar incident happened during the last year of my B.A. with a test in anthropology. This time my mark was a C. Again, I asked a student whose mark was an A if I could read her paper, stating she had such a good mark I thought I could learn from what she had written. She bought it, not noticing the sarcasm in my request and proudly handed it over. I could not make head or tail of the essay. It was all over the place. Actually, it was pathetic. I did not bother confronting the professor, an alcoholic (you could smell the booze on his breath when you went up close to him in class at ten in the morning), and the girl looked and behaved like a slut. Ass-grazing skirts were the style for the first time in history, and some professors had told me that it drove them to distraction when the female students sat in the first row in their classrooms. It was easy to see how this one made the grade. Nowadays, of course, you can't tell the difference between a 'ho and a nice girl, because of the way they dress.

Another time, after knocking on a professor's office door and just walking in, I found a male student sitting on his lap. I was embarrassed, but shocked? No, no more. The rumour was that the professor was homosexual, although he had a wife. He was known to be mean. I had never been one of his targets, but after that day, whenever I ran into him, I could feel hatred emanating from him. He has died since. His obituary was positive.

I don't remember for sure how I learned — I think one of them told me years later — that at the first university I attended, the professors in humanities were terrified I would choose their course. I had the reputation of asking too many questions and often challenged their position on whatever subject they were expounding. Of course, I was their age or older, well-read compared to the younger students, and their authority did not impress me. I can see their point now. At the time it never entered my mind. I was oblivious to their power, my standard of living was often above theirs, and their general culture was very limited. They didn't seem to know anything beyond their particular field of interest, the same as many professionals like doctors, lawyers, and judges I was to meet later. I was so giddy at being a university student that I didn't suspect the hostility and resentment, although when chatting with the professors you could sense they were from a *petit-bourgeois* background.

Shenanigans

There was a Marxist professor — communism had not collapsed yet, and spouting Marxist theory was quite the style then — who used his classes to revile every material comfort enjoyed in our society. He so bad-mouthed capitalism that I figured he was from a working-class background and been very poor at one time. To illustrate his point of view, he described how he once had worked in an aristocratic household in England, where he helped serving guests at the table, and where they would converse in front of the servants as if they did not exist. (Downton Abbey?) You could see that really riled him. I asked him at one point whether, given his ideology, he put his money in the bank like everyone else. He did. Although he had a mistress as well as a wife, he showed an interest in having an affair with me. I kept him interested (I was learning from my younger peers) until after the final exams because I didn't want my marks to go south. I was depending on grants for my tuition. I was sure he was very vindictive and easily humiliated. I was also certain I would eventually — having manipulated him — have to pay for it, but I had no idea when or how retribution would manifest itself. He indeed exacted his revenge when, at the end of my Master's degree, running into him by chance, I confided that my dream was to teach at our university after I received my Ph.D. "I can assure you, you'll never teach here!" he scoffed. This was more or less true: in theory, you couldn't be hired by the same institution where you had studied without having taught in another one first. Nevertheless, I was shattered. His tone indicated rage and will to hurt. I was still naïve enough to think my marks and thesis would count in my favour, since my doctorate would be acquired at a different and more prestigious university, but from that moment my worry about not being able to find a position as professor became a nagging concern.

Nevertheless, I had enjoyed my undergraduate years, because I was learning so much. History 101 was such a pleasure, the professor a real pro (after him, the others, duds). Some classes were just deadly, with the teachers not knowing how to liven up their subject, not being passionate about them. I did not feel out of place with the younger students. Some of the male ones, not realizing my age, shyly attempted to date me. I turned them down gently, telling them how flattered I was. It was nice for my ego, though.

Years later, the Marxist professor's girlfriend became a friend of mine during the period of my first separation from Speedy. She owned a little house near campus and he would visit her there. They had met when she was his student at some college in the U.S. He was one of her thesis supervisors at the time, and when he had been offered a better position at our university, she had simply moved to be near him. No one could understand what she saw in him. He was married, and far from handsome, with a protruding jaw made even worse by the fact that he was always extremely sullen and cranky with a perpetual pout. She had no qualms about telling me that he would always take her from behind, information I had not sought. Perhaps she even meant the anal way; I did not ask any questions. Did it hurt? She had totally been under his spell all those years, but her resolve had begun to crack. She was known to his wife, and by now she had started to believe he would never divorce. I don't know what she was living on. She didn't teach and was getting on in years.

What probably opened her eyes to the futility of investing still more time in the relationship was the fact that when her lover had a heart attack and was confined to a hospital bed, she was not allowed to visit since she was not a family member. I believe his wife, who had closed her eyes to their liaison for all those years, saw to it this rule be strictly observed by the nurses, and thus exacted her revenge as well as sort of officially reinstated her status in that particularly peculiar marriage. It was to be expected. What had not been anticipated was the heart attack.

Another professor made the remark that it had to be stressful for a man to divide himself between two women, running from one household to the other, even if the two females lived in the same part of town. It was a common and ancient arrangement, anthropologically inevitable, since there aren't enough men to go around, males preferring younger women after they've married one more or less their own age. A few years after this reality check, my friend moved to Florida, where she used to visit her parents, and where she now allowed herself to meet a French restaurant owner. They married, but it didn't work out that well. She used to send me Christmas cards and complain of her new life. She could not understand my wanting to leave my husband. I was surprised. She had wished so much for her ex-lover to become free of his spouse. Obviously she was not the feminist she had claimed to be. Perhaps she did not relish the idea of seeing me free, free to meet men, perceiving me subconsciously as a threat.

The judicious if catty remark about a man running himself ragged dividing his life between two households had been made by a professor of geology, whose girlfriend was a pal of the Marxist's mistress. I can't recall how I met that couple; some party or other, I suppose. The geology professor was also married, but separated from his wife, who lived in another city. He could afford to be contemptuous of his unfaithful colleague. But his girlfriend, that's another story. She was most unhappy about not being the legal wife. Years and years later, I ran into her and she asked, "Have you heard the news?" I couldn't think of anything. She gloated that her lover was finally going to make an honest woman out of her (as she put it), and showed me her engagement ring. It was not a diamond, a sapphire, an emerald, a ruby, ersatz or otherwise, I remember that much. It was something opaque. She was so happy. I was glad for her. At the same time, I remembered that the Marxist's mistress had once confided in me that Geology had a very small wienie. My response had been "How did she know?"

It appears they indulged in swinging parties. At that point it came back to me that very soon after I had made his acquaintance, when he was dean of science, Geology had brought me back to his apartment for a reason that sounded legitimate, although we both knew it was just a pretext. There, very much in view, lay a book in French — its original language — by the author whose novels were the subject of my doctoral thesis. I oohed and aahed, of course, especially since I knew his French was not good enough for him to enjoy reading this novel. Clearly, he wanted to impress me so he could bed me. It did not happen. I did not know him well enough. I did not want to do that to his girlfriend, and besides, he did not appeal to me. That sounds strange in the 21st century. At the time, I had no idea they were swingers. I probably would have been shocked. As it was, I ascribed his advances to my being irresistible…! A few years later, as a member of the committee whose final approval determined who was hired as faculty in the various departments, he nixed my application for a position at the university.

During this brief first separation from Speedy, I had a one-night stand at lunchtime with an insurance salesman, a broker, I should say (sounds less tawdry). He was very successful and gorgeous, and his wife was originally from France. They were, for some reason, part of our wider social circle. The people in our town, before so many

French-Canadians artists became famous in the world, did not make the distinction between being French-speaking from France or from Canada. We had been introduced to this couple at a party very soon after we had moved out of Quebec. This "to-die-for," so good-looking insurance peddler pursued me for years, until during this period on my own I relented out of curiosity. It was not a memorable encounter. I was exhausted from the emotional stress of seeing a divorce lawyer, and he had a meeting to go to. It was years after we had first met, and the passion was not there. He certainly was no better lover than my husband. None of them were, actually, in the end. In any case, after this one-time tryst I lost touch with him for years. One day, finally legally separated by then, I ran into him in the farmers' market. I was speechless. He had aged so much. (Hell, our old crowd had always been ten years older than us, and by this point he must have been in his seventies.) "Look at you!" he cried. "How good you look!" I asked about his wife and daughters. They had sold their house and moved to Toronto after he retired. I remembered one particular party when the lady had boasted to the women around her what a wonderful husband he was. This was just five minutes after he had propositioned me. My years of intense socializing taught me the more attentive a man is to his wife, the most likely he is to be cheating on her.

During the 1970s, in the early phase of my graduate studies, we had an invited professor from France who was obviously homosexual (the term "gay" was not used in those days). Interestingly, when I was studying for my Master's I had done research on certain adjectives used in Old French and discovered that the early meaning of that word was to designate such a person. Gays have made that point since.

I loved this professor. His classes were very stimulating. He died a couple of years later of what was believed to be a cancer, sarcoma if I recall correctly. Knowing how sexually active he was, I concluded he suffered from AIDS, which had not yet been discovered when he was alive. A fellow student friend of mine who, under his "guidance," had confirmed his own sexual orientation, concurred. Apparently the professor used to roam certain parks after dark, looking for partners. Fortunately for my friend, they had never engaged in anal or oral sex, although there must have been some hanky-panky going on because the professor was advised by my friend to have a doctor look at his penis. Apparently his foreskin did not pull back. I flirted outrageously with the two of them and they reciprocated. When I learned of his death, I was sorry I would never see him again.

This fellow student, who was in several of my classes, became my buddy except for afterschool hours and on weekends, since I lived out of town. The one-hour driving commute was hellish during rush hour, heroic in winter storms. When I arrived on campus, I would head for the graduate library, where I slept for an hour in an armchair before my first class of the day, having had to get up at 5 a.m. in order to make it for 9 a.m., after studying the whole evening before. This, three days a week. I was on autopilot most of the time anyway, entirely sustained by my drive to change my life when my studies were completed. I did rent an apartment in the city during the last two years of writing my thesis.

One evening, students in a certain course were invited to attend a *soirée* at the home of a couple who were both professors in our department. As people started to depart around one o'clock, they approached my buddy and I and asked if we would stay after the others had left. I was tired and had been bored for quite a while, so I declined, as did my friend, who had gotten a ride with me. Afterward in the car, we wondered what they had found so exceptional about us that they sought our particular company. We hardly knew them. Sometime later I heard they were swingers. Obviously, they thought we were a couple and did not know my friend was gay. They must have found it titillating, that in their minds I was an adulterer. Homosexuals had not started coming out of the closet yet, so if a man and a woman were close they were thought of as a couple. Gossip just thrived in the ivory tower.

At university, a lot of the good-looking guys turned out to be gay. Such was another student I occasionally talked to. I never had any inkling he was not interested in women until we attended the same colloquium in Normandy. At this scholarly gathering, several of the papers were given by various stars of French literary criticism. Roland Barthes, the famous semiotician, a known homosexual, was there, surrounded by a bevy of his *mignons*, students of his. One day after lunch, before the start of the afternoon program, we were all strolling in the gardens of the *chateau* where we were lodged when our paths crossed, Barthes with his court, I, on my own. The great man stopped and gave me a big smile, encouraging me to speak to him, accustomed as he was to being besieged by an army of admirers dying to attract his attention with arcane questions on literary matters. I couldn't think of anything to discuss with him that would be worthy of interrupting their stroll and their pleasure in each other's company, so I just smiled back and continued on my way.

After that, I felt quite at ease in his presence, which led me to attend the nightly get-togethers where wine was served and dance music played. The first night no one paid attention to me, not even my compatriot, and there were very few women present. That in itself was odd. Usually it's the other way around, with the females outnumbering the males. The guys were dancing together. The second night I had to admit to myself that this was an almost strictly gay gathering as I sadly contemplated the pairing off. It dawned on me why my acquaintance had been less than enthusiastic when I told him that I, as he, would be attending the colloquium, why, contrary to my expectation, he had ignored me and not sat with me on the plane, why he had given me the cold shoulder since we had arrived, which had offended me. He was hoping to score and didn't want to encourage me to hang around with him, lest he be taken for a heterosexual. Maybe he was hoping Barthes would fancy him, so he could gain some advantage job-wise as a result. He did get a position as a professor of linguistics right after getting his Ph.D., although his degree was in literature, having bluffed, and what else, his way through. But then, all the young men were always hired.

In any case, I met other people at that conference, one of them a Frenchman with a car who offered to show four of us around the Normandy countryside. We skipped the presentations and went driving with him, visiting places we would not have seen otherwise. The experience was especially thrilling for me since it was the region where my ancestors had come from. That outing is one of the best memories of my university years. It must have been so as well for the man who had invited us, because after I returned home I received an envelope containing a postcard, as is the discreet custom in Europe, commenting on that excursion and thanking me for the joy and pleasure he had gotten out of it. I think it was a first for him, meeting a French-Canadian. I was proud that he had been impressed. I kept the card and its envelope for a long time. It was one of the rare times in my life when I had known happiness. It stands out as such in my mind, in spite of the fact that I had caught a terrible cold on the flight over and felt miserable the whole time I was there. But then I've always caught a cold when traveling overseas. My immune system was weakened by the lack of sleep. Another indelible memory from that trip in Normandy: every morning, bottles of local wine and calvados were on each of the long tables set for our breakfast.

In those days universities were hotbeds, so to speak, of illicit romances, as described in numerous novels. There was another professor, of Italian descent, who as the saying goes, "Fucked anything that walked." I never took one of his courses, but his wife built the last house I shared with my husband. The real estate agent who had brokered the sale was full of admiration for this woman, or rather, her money. She haughtily advised me that the owner did not wish to have anything to do with buyers. One could communicate with the agent only, even after the sale was concluded. There was not to be any meeting between the two parties. According to the broker, it was the history professor's wife's hobby to design and build houses, something to do with her parents having left her a fortune in Montana, and being acquainted with the Marlboro Man. Obviously, the semiotics of an ad bearing the image of a cowboy in a mountainous setting featuring the logo of a cigarette brand did not speak to the agent, who basked in the glory of being associated with someone connected with culture and higher education.

In spite of, or because of, Mrs. Montana being an active patron in the classical music community in our town, she struck me as being a *parvenue*, a *nouvelle riche,* whom her husband, the history professor, had married for her money. I was very tempted to tell the agent about his philandering, so annoyed was I at her awe of Mrs. Montana, who I thought had the elegance of a cleaning woman on the job, according to a photo I was shown where she leaned on her grand piano clad in what looked like a house-dress, clashing with the classiness of the musical instrument. I surmised the lady had married the professor because of the prestige of being associated with academe. She turned a blind eye to his running around.

By coincidence, she and I shared the same cleaning woman, who had mentioned to me this client of hers with tons of money, who had built an extraordinary house with a room for recitals, with sculptures in the garden, and who was so busy with the arts that she had no time to lift a finger, housekeeping-wise. Her home was filthy.

I had occasion years later to attend one of the recitals, after which I asked to visit the home. The husband, who was hovering around, offered himself as guide and as soon as we reached the kitchen he started nuzzling me in the neck, thus confirming his reputation as a letch. I backed away promptly. He had no idea who I was. In the early nineties, while traveling through Turkey, I thought of him because his name was the same as a certain region in that country. The poor sod has died since. I wonder if she went back to Montana. I know she came to my house after we moved in, being sure we were at work, and marveled to the agent about my good taste in decorating it. It was a house she had built for fun, custom-made with the best materials. It was her baby, but she never lived there. Because it was so different, it was not easy to sell and had been on the market for two years. Unconventional in its exterior and with such a big open space inside, it scared prospective buyers away. They did not notice the perfection, the care that had been put into building it, but the moment I stood inside the house (which I was viewing out of curiosity), in my imagination my belongings started falling into place inside the various rooms. I had to have it. It was contemporary, in the middle of the city, and close to my work. My reasoning was that since my husband refused to move to Toronto, which had more to offer as far as my interests were concerned, then I would get to live in a house that really appealed to me. My husband resisted the idea of change at first, but after a while he acquiesced and fell in love with it as well.

Acquiring the Ph.D.

The years of writing my doctoral thesis were a lonely and desperate business. Lonely, because the research has to be more or less unique, and in the case of my chosen subject I sensed my supervisor's lack of interest — he had never read the author in question; the other two readers on the committee were also indifferent to my project of showing similarities between my chosen writer's themes and the tenets of Nietzsche's philosophy. In my case writing the thesis was also a desperate business because of the ensuing lack of support and the uncertainty of reaching my ultimate goal. I thought it would be a good idea to submit some chapters for comments to a visiting professor, a compatriot and contemporary of mine, familiar with my author's work. How naïve and foolish of me! This professor was an ex-priest, who as a still practicing Catholic, had probably never read the German philosopher and, no doubt, from Nietzsche's reputation alone held him to be a veritable Anti-Christ. His was a totally unexpected and vicious reaction. Tact did not enter into it. There was no softening of the blow: bristling with hostility, he flatly stated the comparison I was attempting couldn't be made, declared it preposterous. He even urged me to abandon the entire project. I could feel his rage at my bold pretension to find common ground between a writer stemming from French-Canadian Catholic society and the nihilist who claimed that God is dead. As an individual steeped in the close-minded faith of the Church, he obviously couldn't stomach what I was doing. I suspect what rattled him the most with such a notion was that it came from a woman. Had I been a male student, I'm sure my work would have met with his approval, or at least his encouragement for tackling such a difficult and original project. I had been counting on him to arouse some enthusiasm in my supervisors. I was heartbroken and stunned by his rebuttal, completely devastated for quite a while, as if I had lost someone dear. My ever present anguish reached new depths. What to do? How could this be? Was I supposed to dump the product of years of labour and start on something else? After a while, I was able to see through his attitude and rallied. I was not going to be defeated. I would show them. Resilience.

This experience with the defrocked one left me uneasy about my oral defense. The academic world, at least in those days, was staunchly misogynistic. Women professors were paid less than men, and perhaps still are. Would the examiners resent what I had accomplished, and fail me? There were to be five of them: the one supervisor, the two readers, another professor from our department, and one from yet another department (in my case, naturally, philosophy). None had ever read my novelist (even my head supervisor couldn't be bothered because the writer was not from France, which was in a way insulting, but such was the snotty attitude in that environment, where racism flourished, as well as sexism. I was the object of both; however, not being the victim type, I chose to ignore the discrimination). The five professors on the panel had to examine my work carefully to see if it held together and I had proven my point. Would they question the very premise my thesis was based on, as had the ex-priest, although my supervisors had let me carry on? As it turned out, they accepted what I was trying to say with very little criticism. I even sensed some muted admiration. One of them felt the need to mention some point I should have touched on and hadn't. Out of 400 pages, which were very tightly and logically organized, they had to find at least one thing wrong.

I had worked myself into such a state preparing for this defense that the whole event played over and over in my mind for days afterward. I couldn't shake it, I couldn't control it, it was totally beyond my will. The adrenaline rush for the fight I expected this last hurdle to be, following the years of intensive research and writing, as well as the other obstacles I had faced along the way, was so great that after I finally was granted the Ph.D. I thought I would collapse. Truth be told, it appears the powers that be didn't give a shit one way or the other. In fields that weren't exact science, they passed anyone who managed to actually finish a thesis. I know, because I read the doctoral dissertation of a friend who graduated the same year as I did in literature, and also that of a professor in my field. Both works were verbiage. They were never published, and neither were the theses of my fellow students. Being younger, most of them were nevertheless hired by universities. They would use snippets of those works as the basis for presentations and articles under various titles, rehashing the same stuff over and over again, building up their C.V.s that way. That's how the game was played, and they had no qualms about it. It's not something that came to me naturally.

The Search

Because I was so desperate to be offered an academic position, I subsequently concentrated on submitting my work to various university presses for publishing. It took me one year to rewrite the thesis toward that purpose. It was accepted by a prestigious institution, and when the book came out two years after I graduated, it received nothing but favorable reviews, no criticism. Ironically, the press which published it hails from the same university where that visiting professor, the defrocked priest who so reviled my work, was teaching at the time. The gratifying reviews confirmed my opinion that spite had been the major source of his animosity. After my book came out, I received phone calls at home from a couple of lecturers in literature thanking me for having made those particular novels the object of my research. There being a dearth of published studies on the subject, they were grateful because my book was a great help to them in covering this novelist's work in their courses. This writer's use of words is so extravagant and unusual that his first book was rejected by all the

French language publishing firms this side of the Atlantic. It was finally accepted by a famous house in Paris, and the rest is history. Unfortunately, the novels are not translatable due to the style, which relies heavily on wordplay, leading to multiple levels of meaning. This recognition from those who were actually using my work confirmed the fact that I had produced something substantial, worthy, and unique in my field, but that gave me no comfort. I had failed in my quest for a professorship. I was sitting at home while the fruit of my labor toward such a goal was helping those who had been my rivals in competing for positions at the very time I was being interviewed for those positions.

One of those interviews had taken place on the west coast, thousand of miles across the country. It was February and snowing very hard, with heavy, wet flakes, when normally in that benign climate flowers should have been coming out. I was dressed for spring when I should have been wearing snow boots. I traipsed around campus soaked and chilled to the bone. The people I met did not seem to notice my discomfort. I guess they figured since I came from winter country, I wasn't bothered by this unseasonable weather. I remember, with embarrassment now, taking off my dripping socks in the French Department chairman's office and laying them out on top of the radiator to dry. According to someone I told the story to sometime later, that move did not help my case. It was a stupid thing to do, but nervousness and extreme eagerness and earnestness made me take leave of my senses. They also requested I teach a language class while I would be observed by a couple of professors. It was unexpected, and I was totally unprepared. It had not happened in previous job interviews. It felt like a trap. My field was literature, not grammar.

They asked me to show them how I would teach the subjunctive. Without looking into it beforehand, I had no idea. I floundered, feeling as if I was drowning. I did not get the position. It was mentioned I had no methodology. My having published did not count for anything. I had a feeling they were getting pleasure in seeing me fail, as if they had already made up their minds. Perhaps it had to do with the fact I was a married woman. I did state I would relocate, but honest to a fault, I let them know my husband would not give up his job to follow me to the ends of the earth. Very callous of me, to be willing to live away from him. The reverse would have been acceptable, due to the double standard. Being males and putting themselves in my husband's place, they figured trouble would ensue in the marriage from this situation, which would then affect my professional life. Well, trouble there had been forever in large part due to Speedy's own absences. It was my turn. I should have simply lied and stated my spouse was ready to move with me. I've learned since that's how you play the game. Once you're in, you do what you want. Inertia is on your side.

The same scenario more or less unfolded on the east coast, where the chairwoman assured me she wanted me badly for the advertised position. Of course, it depended on the hiring committee's decision. Had I been male, it would have played differently. Indeed, in every position I applied for the chosen candidate turned out to be a young man, often gay, whom the women interviewers favored because for females, homosexual men were so pleasant to have around and there was no competition, sexually speaking. As for male interviewers — many of them gay themselves, outed or not — they either perceived the young men as potential objects of desire, members of the same oppressed community, or if heterosexuals, as individuals they could bond with professionally without sexual tension entering into the relationship. Unless they are Don Juans, straight males do not relish having an attractive female around who is out of bounds. They find it distracting. One explanation I was given for this trend of favoring young, unattached males was that they were more pliable and deserved to be given the chance to start a career, as opposed to a woman who had a husband who could support her. So much for excellence! And how ironic: I desperately needed such employment to achieve financial independence, which would have made me, in their eyes, a more deserving candidate.

Shaky Teaching

Upon receiving my diploma, I was offered a language teaching position in a satellite campus, considered the lowest status possible in a literature department, not worthy of a post-graduate candidate since such courses exist outside academe, not necessarily requiring an advanced university degree of the teacher. I felt humiliated that in spite of my thesis being accepted for publication, I had not been offered a position in my specialty. I was very despondent. Since I had no formal training in teaching French as a foreign language, I lacked confidence, which added to my dejection. Besides, I was physically exhausted. The students could sense my vulnerability and incompetence. Some of the females were merciless, while the males were more indulgent. That first semester was a disaster, a nightmare. The years of juggling family and studies, out of town, had caught up with me.

During the Christmas holidays I was in a car accident which prevented me from going back to my lecturer's duties. My contract was not renewed in the spring. I expected as much, but it came as a blow. Without any leverage, in a pathetic effort to salvage my dream of a university career, I confronted the chairman of the hiring committee, who was ever so pleased to tell me I had had very bad evaluations from the students. I believe this guy was a medievalist. No sympathy at all for a married woman who was seeking emancipation, when she should be home, wearing a chastity belt, waiting on/for her husband. He was downright hostile. I could sense he felt I should never have had access to his world. I applied to and was turned down by community colleges, where anyone who held a Ph.D. was resented and punished for having reached that level. I answered ads for office jobs in the city, hoping to keep my little apartment and preserve some aspects of my life there, but I was unsuccessful. "Overqualified" was the unanimous response, even when I pretended I only had a high school diploma. They all told me "You wouldn't be happy here." I didn't give the impression I was an office person, although I tried, and had started looking for such a job even before receiving my degree. I gave up, moved my furniture from the apartment to the family basement, and started transforming my thesis into a book for publication. Paring down my doctoral work took me a good year and kept my mind from freefalling into emptiness after the arcane, intellectual stimulation I had grown accustomed to.

I no longer had any contact with that community which had been my world for so long. I had severed all ties with our former social circle, my studies being a priority, and I found I had no longer anything in common with housewives. My being an older married woman had prevented my fellow students in graduate school from perceiving me as one of their peers. The females thought I was an odd duck, the males regarded me with suspicion, and I did feel duty-bound to go home and be with my husband every weekend. I would have loved to find a close circle of friends at university, and break all ties with my former life, but my only buddy during my doctoral years was gay. None of my professors attracted me. They were all shocked anyway, at my having an apartment in town. They were convinced it was for philandering purposes. They had no idea what the rush hours were like driving between my hometown and the big city, or through winter storms along the lake. Acute despair is counterproductive. My reputation of being a liberated woman might well have been transmitted by code in the letters of recommendation I brought with me to the various interviews I was granted regarding advertised positions in my field, and it might have negatively affected my chances of being hired. After all, academe had turned out to be the second most misogynistic community I have encountered, after the Church. Because of the quality of my scholarly work, that I still could be discriminated against never occurred to me at the time. Probably because of being in denial, but after I found another career, I put two and two together. Paglia *et al* are younger than me and were never subjected to the censure and rejection I suffered.

I typed my book myself on an electric machine, not knowing how to use a computer, and I never thought of getting one. After a few minor corrections, it was published. It had a beautiful red cover. I proudly brought a copy to my cancerous, cantankerous mother in the hospital. She brushed the book away with her hand, refusing to look at it, and smirked, "What was the point of all that labor? What are you going to do with it? What a waste of time!" No doubt she was angry I had accomplished at age fifty what she had been dead set against when I was sixteen, but I was not prepared for such a mean reaction. I expected her illness to have mellowed her. Instead, it felt as if she hated me. On another visit, the lady who shared her room exclaimed upon our being introduced, "But she's not fat! You said this daughter was fat." After that, I closed my heart, accepting the fact I never had had a mother, and lost all feelings toward her. She, who had never really lived, was terrified of death and fought it for another six years.

Two years after graduating with my Ph.D., I was offered a seasonal (temporary, in other words) contract ($8,000 for nine months) to replace a professor who was taking a maternity leave at a university about a three-hour drive from where I lived. That position was made available to me on the strength of my by now published thesis, which everyone agreed was brilliant. The chairman was very gracious, in dire need of a last minute replacement, even flirtatious, and I sensed he liked me until I was stupid enough to offer him my book to read. He did, and he never spoke to me again after that. Clearly my work was more scholarly than he had expected, and worse, from a woman he was attracted to. He was probably offended by my liberated stance, which wholly embraced my novelist's unconventional form and style as well as the iconoclastic content of his work, which turned every received idea on its head. My analysis, consisting of a solid deconstruction of the writing, must have hit a nerve, not to mention the considerable skill deployed in accomplishing such a study no other literary theorist had managed where this author was concerned, and shaken him, since this professor never published anything (at least during the time I was there).

At that time, many of the people who sat on hiring committees did not hold doctorates. They had been recruited in the early sixties, when there was a dearth of experts in French literature in North America. Universities had money for the humanities then. I had a good relationship with everyone else on staff, although we lecturers were clearly exploited as seasonal workers. I was constantly weary, what with my commuting by train for six hours every weekend, back and forth between my home and my rented digs, and the constant worry about finding another position at the end of my contract, in addition to living on a student budget in the basement of a lady dwarf's house, which did not feature a kitchen sink. Although I had a car, I walked quite a distance to campus every day, ending up with thick calluses under my feet. That's when I purchased my first backpack. I'm still using it. In retrospect, I concede I could have spent my whole meager wages on living more comfortably, but I was determined to put money aside toward my future liberation from married life. I led a very Spartan and solitary existence, and none of my colleagues were in the same circumstances.

Published and Perished

I knew my husband tremendously resented the fact that I was not living in our home during the week. In addition to being deprived of my services when he happened to be there, my working so far away was not something he could explain at the company, where no one had a clue how the academic world operates. Even to me, it really made sense, in as much as I thought I was working toward putting together a reasonable C.V., but it generated a great deal of tension in my life, since the necessity of going home every weekend sapped my energy and enthusiasm toward participating in extracurricular activities, such as departmental meetings, where various tasks would be assigned to faculty. My apparent lack of interest in cooperating, fostered by the fact that at my meager salary, I felt doing anything extra was participating in my own exploitation, could have influenced the chair in opposing the renewal of my contract a third time, after granting me a second year when another female professor became pregnant. I should have shown more subservience and made myself indispensable when it came to doing the Joe-jobs a department head likes to foist on lecturers who are hoping for tenure. I was told that had my contract been renewed three years in a row, the university legally exposed itself to having to offer me a tenure track position. That information was a terrible blow, but neither was I convinced of its veracity. After all, I had published a book with incredible reviews which was more than a lot of other entrenched lecturers and professors had done. Someone else in the hiring committee did not want me around, but why? After my years as a student, I had learned it was best to keep to myself, and quiet, so as not to attract attention. Besides, the former department chairman, who had been so upset with my book, had now been replaced by a woman, so I could not figure out whom I had displeased.

Later I understood that I had inadvertently reopened the wounds of a scandal in the department. Near the end of my second term, when it became obvious to me that this time my contract would not be renewed, I asked a colleague against whom I had mysteriously been warned (backstabbing flourishes in that environment), who had doggedly tried to befriend me, and from whom I finally accepted a dinner invitation at her home. I asked this colleague why so-and-so, who was so nice to me, disliked her so much. After much hesitation, she agreed to tell me if I swore I would not mention it to anyone. I learned that so-and-so, whom this friendly colleague knew hated her, had been previously married to another professor in the department. This man had had an affair with another male professor who happened to be a friend of the colleague with whom I was dining that evening. There had been a messy divorce, and apparently so-and-so, who hated her for knowing what had been going on (the same-sex liaison), thought no one else in the department was aware of the matter. Shortly after I had been apprised of this affair at my colleague's home, the betrayed "ex-wife," with whom I had been friends, started giving me the cold shoulder. She must have suspected I had been told of her humiliation.

This so-and-so was also the coordinator of studies in the language section of the department, and she did not teach literature. In one of my language classes, I had a student who did not show up for the final exam. He sent me a note saying he had fallen down the stairs at his lodgings that morning and was unable to walk. I duly reported this development to the coordinator and she explained that this particular student was, out of fear, incapable of bringing himself to write exams, and that he always appealed to her to excuse him. She did because he was so sweet — always a little gift for her — and she let him pass from year to year. Sensing my shock and disapproval at this disturbing news, she assured me this year she would be firm and not let him get away with it. Some days later I was at the receptionist's desk when a bouquet of flowers arrived and so-and-so was paged to receive it. I looked at the name of the sender. When she picked up the bouquet she defiantly looked at me and said nothing. She knew I had made the connection.

That episode was, I think, the kiss of death for me as far as my contract being renewed. So-and-so, in the meantime, since parting with her homosexual husband, had become engaged to yet another professor in the department, a widower. Both of them were on the hiring committee, something I always thought was not allowed, for obvious ethical reasons. This pair together, with the present chairwoman (whom I should have buttered up during the last year but hadn't), voted against rehiring me. I suspect the chairwoman because in April, as my contract was to expire, she saddled me with supervising the Master's dissertation of a student who was an absolute lost cause. No one else had been willing to undertake this task, the young man a pathetic nullity. I accepted because, hoping against all hope, I thought it would turn the tide regarding the renewal of my contract. It didn't. Disgusted, I never again made the trip back to that institution after May. I never found out if that young man got his degree.

So ended my attempts at achieving a university career. I fell into the worst depressive state I had ever experienced, and I had been through many bouts. I stopped eating because I couldn't swallow. The food would not go down past my throat. I was overcome by panic attacks and anxiety so fierce I was paralyzed when faced with the most trivial decisions. I could not concentrate enough to read or watch television, being unable to sit still. My insomnia raged. In terminal despair, not seeing any solution to filling the void, assuaging that incessant gnawing inside me, I saw a psychiatrist who specialized in hypnotism. It didn't work. I was too tense to let go, beyond reach. We got to talking, however, especially about him. Finally, the easy way out for him in my case was to pronounce there are no bad situations, only bad reactions to situations. He was Jewish, so, in utter frustration, I told him concentration camps weren't bad then, that the Jews just reacted badly to them. He was nonplussed, and agreed my problems were beyond his expertise. In my opinion, what makes people unhappy is the frustration, rage, and the feeling of helplessness of not having control over their own lives, the degree of misery depending on what you imagine your life should be. My present cleaning woman is thrilled to be paid good money for what she does, and in being autonomous. After all, she does not have training for anything else. The benefits of positive reaction apply mostly to physical pain. You can really make it ten times worse by being hysterical about it. Some people dearly hang on to their ailments, solely in order to get attention and feel important.

That was never my attitude. In order to get myself out of the house and tame the anguish, I started doing volunteer work. At first I accompanied cancer patients in the ambulance on their way to various treatments. Little did I know what further ordeals the future had in store for me. As an activity, I found it unchallenging. One poor soul I was assigned to could not control his foul flatulence when I would sit or walk beside him on his stretcher. I did not mind, but it embarrassed him tremendously. I could see he'd rather I was not there, or would have preferred the help of a male instead. My company was doing him more harm than good. I felt badly for him. I switched to working in the hospital library twice a week, sorting donated paperbacks and making the rounds with a cart through the various wards, offering or collecting our reading material. There were two other women volunteers attending with me. I remember making a remark about saving money for my future — I was by then fifty-one — and one of them replied "You have a future?" Besides the fact that in those days fifty was old, it was inconceivable to her my life would be other than what it was at that moment, until I died. Yet in my mind I was still dreaming of one day leaving my marriage, although I had no prospects of earning a living, and knew with absolute certainty that my husband would never consent to paying alimony, which meant engaging into a protracted, toxic battle. My familial tremors rendered worse by the chronic insomnia and increasing with age as well, coupled with the occasional involuntary movements which accompanied them, precluded me from typing fast enough and faultlessly. Office work was out of the question, as it had been in my twenties, hence my marriage was a roof over my head and food to eat. Should I have become a salesclerk or a factory worker?

Portrait of a Husband

The best way to describe my ex is that he was a mathematical genius, a master at fixing anything of a mechanical, electrical, plumbing or automotive nature, very resourceful and patient, never panicking in any tricky situation which could throw me in a frenzy. He was also fearless, at least in his car. Once, going up a snowy hill where such vehicles were not allowed — we were taking the kids tobogganing — I, warning him not to (which in itself was enough to spur him on) drove along a cliff on our right side, and inevitably the car slid sideways. The ledge of snow resting on a void started to give way under the weight, and Speedy very, very carefully, not losing his cool, managed to back all the way down the rutted incline while I envisioned us tumbling over the edge, breaking our necks. Another time, as Speedy was driving an RV too fast on a skiing trip in the mountains up north, with signs urging drivers not to use the icy roads, the vehicle slipped on the ice and ended up with its front wheels hanging over a precipice. Again we escaped our predicament in one piece, and with no damage to the vehicle. The people who rescued us thought we were idiots. That made me just as angry as the fear I had felt. I myself would never have exposed myself or the children to such danger, but my husband loved that kind of challenge. He had to show he could control anything, obsessed about being the winner in any situation he found himself in.

Numero Uno

Speedy resented everything I was, had, or had accomplished, forever making me pay for it. To be fair, all men of my generation (that's the operative word here) I subsequently met turned cold when they found out about my degrees and my position in the judiciary. They were bothered, felt threatened, and became hostile. Especially when physically attracted to me. It was as if I was tricking them with my sex appeal. On the other end, some of them were turned off immediately if, not having yet met me in person, I advised them over the phone that my hair was gray. That was a test I secretly put them through, my reasoning being that if a male was not sure enough of himself to be seen with an aging female, then he was not worth bothering with. Of

163

course, some of them dye their hair too. If only they knew how much more sexy and attractive they would be if they let it go silver. I believe my own natural, now almost–white, crowning glory has a lot to do with the oh-so-heartwarming flattering remarks (at my age) I frequently get. How did it come to that? I wish I had known how things would turn out when, growing up, I was treated as an ugly duckling. It was so disheartening.

I finally left Speedy after thirty-six years of marriage and two previously failed attempts to do so. I could never go near my husband and express mere tenderness by simply touching him. It was always taken as an invitation to fuck. I felt continually thwarted in my desire for warmth and closeness. His attitude led me to repress any affectionate gesture toward him. I didn't relish being uniquely an object of sexual gratification, as was the wife in the movie *Angela's Birthday Party*. Speedy had this maddening habit of grabbing my breasts when my hands were plunged in hot water doing the dishes. It was cute and endearing in the first years of togetherness, but just annoying after years of marital strife. The few times I did refuse his advances altogether (up until the last two years of our union), he would get so angry and bully me for the rest of the day. I soon realized it would be easier for me to go along with him immediately. After twenty years, when feminism was well implanted, I came to view this forced copulating as rape. On the subject of rape, it is Marilyn French, I believe, who said, "Men rape women with their eyes." Islamists know this for a fact: that is why they insist their women hide their whole bodies under a burqa or a niqab, so that other men cannot carry the image of those same women in their fantasies, thus having their way with them and owning them.

The fact that I experienced pleasure whenever my husband and I had intercourse did not mean that I wanted to do it whenever the mood struck him — which was every time he looked at me — just that I had a strong sense of duty and that I realized I was lucky to still be so strongly desired by my spouse while aging like everyone else. I was afraid of displeasing him, but giving into his sexual appetite made me feel I had absolutely no control over my life. It was not until a couple of years before we finally split up that I denied him his conjugal rights. After we separated and I went to live in an apartment, he found a substitute within a couple of weeks to assuage his robust and pressing sexual needs. I know a man whose wife died of breast cancer after seven years of remission, with three grown-up children, who started dating within two months of his becoming a widower. It does not seem to matter who the date is, as long as it is not a prostitute or an immigrant factory worker. It'll literally do the trick.

Speedy's horniness also translated into prurience in his speech in my presence, whether we were alone or in company. I don't know if he talked dirty with other people, but in front of me he constantly made lewd remarks or crude sexual jokes at the most inappropriate times and totally out of context, especially when I was talking or relating something that put me in a good light. Had he done that with a female co-worker or subordinate, it would have been construed as sexual harassment. Since he has apparently reprised that behaviour with one of our daughters-in-law, a handsome, classy, educated, intelligent woman, I suspect his subconscious motivation for doing so is the same as it was with me. It was one more way for him to torment me, to put me in my place, because as an accomplished female

I posed a threat. Whenever I would be telling him about something that happened to me at work in my capacity as a judge, he would turn it into a joke, thus minimizing the importance of my position, and doing so demeaning me. It was impossible for me to confide in him. If I mentioned problems or difficulties encountered at work, he would immediately start dictating the line of conduct I should follow, without knowing the intricacies of the situation. I was not asking for advice. I just wanted someone to lend me an ear. When a man I released on bail subsequently went on a murder spree, then was himself shot to death by the police, I was crucified in the media. Although those in the know agreed that I only followed the guidelines for the release of an accused person, Speedy became very angry that I followed the advice of the lawyer who was representing me at the coroner's inquest, insisting I should listen to him instead. He was annoyed that this lawyer phoned me every day and kept me apprised of what was happening.

In addition to his sexual aggressiveness, Speedy systematically questioned or opposed any decision or plan of mine regarding the household, an aspect of our common life he absolutely was not the least bit interested in. It's as if he had this drive, this dedication, to make sure I would not get the upper hand, opposing me on principle. Whereas other husbands will agree to take it upon themselves to do certain chores (cutting the grass, washing exterior windows, or just buying certain necessary pieces of furniture), he had to be asked, begged, and finally nagged into it. I purchased a new deck chair, one that had different reclining positions, and had been very difficult to match with the rest of the existing set. He angrily objected that it was too expensive, that its back was not high enough. I told him I'd take it back, so that he could get the chair he liked himself. He never found one. The painter hired to do interior walls was awed to hear that I had to submit my choice of colors to my husband for approval. As far as the trade man was concerned, that was a wife's prerogative. One cleaning woman had the same reaction about my not making decisions on purely domestic trivia which could not possibly concern him. If I said to one of the boys "You need a haircut," Speedy would interfere: "No, you don't really need one."

I felt constantly undermined, and, like the children, poor. At the time of our marriage, my spouse had a relatively low paying job, and while the boys were growing up we had little money, his position in the company having not reached the status he was to achieve later as an executive. To compound the constraints where his small salary kept me, my determination at being a perfect housewife drove me to be extremely thrifty. Waste of any kind was and still is abhorrent to me. I remained the deprived individual I had always been. We had moved to an upscale neighborhood, but our furniture was still the same shabby pieces we had been transferring from house to house since our marriage. He did not see the contradiction. He was proud of living amongst the well-to-do. It attested to his success. The inside of the house was not important to him, and there was no money for that. It bothered me to have an expensive home with an interior that did not match. Similarly, the boys felt like paupers at the local school, attended by the three sons of our immediate neighbors of identical age whose father was a famous medical researcher at the local hospital and whose lifestyle reflected that status. Speedy traveled extensively on business, staying in the best hotels, eating at the best restaurants, with the alcohol flowing, on an expense account before austerity set in and corporations tightened their belts.

Those were elating moments for a man who came from a deprived environment, but they meant misery for us. One trip after another, he was strutting his stuff, money was no object, and his home life was receding far behind. He would fly into a rage whenever I complained of neglect. I envied him, of course. I would not have, if his absences had at least been compensated by extra wealth trickling down to the family, but his good life was due to the expense account, not increases in salary. What galled me the most was that he was not in sales, obliged to travel, but simply a member of an association which set standards worldwide, and he represented the industry. He could easily have passed on some of their meetings, as did some of his colleagues, for whom they were mostly a waste of time, not worth traveling long distances for. Speedy felt no obligation to be with us. He had no qualms about being on the other side of the world for Easter, for example, which deeply offended me because this was to me a holyday on the same scale as Christmas, to be spent within one's family, as I tearfully told him while he was packing. To no avail. I was nothing but a nag. "See you later."

When I came home from my cancer surgery, he, as usual, had a trip planned for that week. I didn't care anymore. Perhaps I was just so happy and relieved the doctor had declared there was no need for treatments. When Speedy asked if I'd be all right on my own, I told him to go ahead with his business, that I'd manage. There were no children left at home, and I'd already been up and around when he was at work. None of my relatives had seen fit to come take care of me. While he was away, his boss phoned to talk to him about something in the middle of the day, not finding him at work. I informed him Speedy was out of town, realizing the man was not aware I had been operated for cancer. Once more it was driven home that my husband didn't consider what happened to his wife important enough to talk about with his co-workers. Shortly after this conversation with Speedy's superior, I received a beautiful bouquet of flowers from him and his wife, delivered at the house since they had not known I had been hospitalized.

Other men in the business often told me they did not travel if they could help it. They only did when it absolutely necessary for their work because they disliked unfamiliar surroundings. The real reason Speedy sought those trips was that they gave him the opportunity to drink compulsively every night in the company of another individual with a similar love of booze. This other alcoholic was an obese creature whom one evening I watched drink scotch after scotch with his dinner, on one occasion when the wives were invited. I was shocked that it was not at least wine. My husband matched him glass for glass. Another time when the better-halves were part of a trip to a city in the U.S. where the women's program mostly consisted of visits to museums and botanical gardens, we came back to the hotel for lunch. The men, who had been at a seminar all morning, were sitting at an outdoor bar. I went up to say hello to Speedy. He said "Hi" and then turned back to the other men and resumed conversation with them, as if I was not standing there. He simply ignored me. I caught the eye of one of his colleagues, whose dismayed look let me know he understood how I felt. He said a few words to me so I wouldn't be left feeling like an intruder.

On those trips where the wives were present, several of the men would take off with their female companions and forget about the scheduled business meetings at the request of their spouses. Those husbands did not for anything want to suffer the consequences of displeasing their wives. To hell with the firm. That was not the case with Speedy. He couldn't have cared less how I felt. He would ask why the long face, and I would tell him, and then he would change the subject. Eventually I stopped accompanying him on those trips after a particular incident which demonstrated that I would be much happier staying at home than traveling with him. Because of his fondness for alcohol, he was always the last one to leave any gathering where it was served. When the wives of other men said it was time to leave, they just complied, setting their glasses down and leaving without argument.

Speedy had promised many times that the moment I stated I was tired and wanted to go back to the room, he would do so. This particular evening, around midnight, I indicated to him it was time to leave. He agreed but added, "You go ahead, I'll come up in five minutes. I'm in the middle of something here." He was always in the middle of something because when he drank he took the floor, dominating the conversation so that others couldn't put a word in edgewise; arguing, mostly. If they did argue, they were harangued, and very loudly at that. My husband got a fix of adrenaline out of confrontation. I left the party and went back to the room, got ready for bed, and then got into bed. Time passed; no husband. Finally, around 2 a.m., he came in in such an inebriated state he was practically crawling on all fours. He flattened on the floor. I could see he wouldn't be able to climb into bed until he had sobered up. This, from a man who had promised to pay attention to my wishes of staying sober and by my side like all the other husbands. I started screaming my fury at him, but he was too drunk to respond other than to grunt, and then he could only whimper because I lost it. I kicked him and kicked him in the ribs with all my might until my rage was spent. The next morning he could hardly walk. When his colleagues asked what was wrong, he explained he had fallen in the bathtub. He ached, but I felt no remorse. I still don't. His co-workers believed him, and smirked, knowing the amount of booze he had ingested the night before. At this gathering, after I had left the room, as he later attempted to explain, he had started on Bailey's Irish Cream on top of the several scotches he had already consumed. Mixing drinks being deadly, especially for him, it was quite plausible he had fallen taking a shower and injured himself. I never accompanied him on a trip after that incident. We also ceased going to parties. Our social life as a couple was over.

Before Family Law Reform

During the thirty-six years I was married to Speedy, I twice attempted to leave him. The first time, in the 1970s, I went to see the only lawyer I knew of without telling him. He was a member of our wider social circle. I had met him at parties, but we weren't friends with the couple. Upon my first appointment with him, I could see he couldn't quite place me. I mentioned we had met before and explained why I had come to him. This was a momentous step in my life and I was very nervous. I was not there on a whim or to fool around. The lawyer was married, but had a reputation with women. Still, I expected him to take me seriously, but he immediately assumed that my reason for wanting to leave my husband was because he was running around. Perhaps because he was himself. I could not persuade him it was because I could not stand my life anymore, that Speedy and I had real irreconcilable differences. He stated mental cruelty was impossible to prove in court and that it could only work if adultery was proven. I assured him Speedy was not unfaithful. He dismissed my denials and suggested we hire a private detective to get evidence of my husband's alleged infidelities. It was sordid, like acting in a B movie, and it made me sick. But since it seemed the only way I could convince the lawyer that adultery was not the reason I wanted to leave my husband, I reluctantly agreed, disgusted.

The idea of spying on someone filled me with shame. In the meantime, the lawyer kept asking me if I would go out to dinner with him. I could not believe he could not see how distressed I was. I was devastated. Dallying with him was the last thing on my mind. His advances made me realize all he was interested in was taking advantage of the situation. Very discouraging. How could I trust this man to have my well-being at heart? He was not about to work hard on my case. Hiring a P.I. was taking the easy way out. Family law had not been reformed yet to include "no-fault" divorce. Unless my lawyer found the right arguments to convince the judge, I would get very little alimony. I knew Speedy would fight tooth and nail to fork out as little as possible. No gentleman, he, especially when humiliated. I phoned the lawyer a couple of times to find out if the P.I. had found anything incriminating. He had nothing. Then, Speedy had a business trip to take. If he had a girlfriend, it was surmised he would take her with him. After he had presumably boarded the plane, I received a phone call from the investigator. He said, "I shouldn't be telling you this, but you're wasting your time and your money. All this guy is interested in is his work. He's married to his job. Besides, I'm not going to risk my life trying to keep up with him following him in my car. I've never seen anyone drive so fast. Believe me, and I know what I'm talking about. Your husband is crazy, but he's not a cheater." Well, I knew that all along. I was relieved that aspect of the proceedings was over, but it wouldn't help my case, considering my lawyer would now lose face. Indeed, he advised me to forget about the whole thing, so I dropped the idea. The entire episode had emotionally exhausted me, and without any support I lacked the courage to pursue the matter. I would have had to find another attorney without any certainty things would turn out any better. The fact that I was acting surreptitiously behind Speedy's back had made it even harder. That particular lawyer was later appointed judge in family court. His wife had left him. He of course found another woman. As a magistrate he was very cranky and feared. He pretended he did not recognize me whenever I ran into him in the courthouse. Maybe my face meant absolutely nothing to him. A selective memory is the best way to salvage one's pride. I myself was very careful to ignore him so as not to have to dwell on one more painful period in my life.

Other Men

Some years later I made a second attempt at leaving my husband, but this time I told him about it, hoping he would leave the house. I knew if he stayed it would make things very difficult, since he would never accept I was not happy in the marriage and there was a need to do something about it. He would also treat me exceptionally kindly in order to weaken my resolve and probably succeed, since I had no one to turn to. He refused to go live somewhere else. Fortunately, he embarked on a long business trip overseas during that time. I was in turmoil nevertheless. I was still in my forties, and I couldn't picture myself without a man in my life. I thought I deserved to be loved. I connected with all the men who had previously conspicuously lusted for me. I had one-night stands with some of them. They acted flattered, but they were most likely frightened when I told them I had left my husband. They could see much clearer than me that my sudden interest in them was a rebound thing, an act of desperation, really. They were mostly all professors. One was moving to the west coast in a few months, and was not about to give up a long time dream for me. Another, who drove a Jaguar XKE, the same model as ours (my excuse to approach him), was offended when I questioned his old-fashioned method in literary criticism. Very tactful of me! His sexual performance was adequate but very perfunctory. All my temporary lovers thought my motivation was sexual starvation, whereas, given the circumstances, like a true female I was longing for emotional and financial security. I was extremely tense during those encounters and got no joy out of them.

In any case, the second divorce lawyer, a no-nonsense type, shared the first one's attitude as far as being successful in getting a judge to order decent support from my husband. Family law hadn't changed and without proof of adultery, my case was weak. Since my husband did not beat me and was a successful executive, this attorney could not understand why I should want to leave him. If I insisted in pursuing the matter, he was confident Speedy would come around and agree to alimony like any humane husband with means would. I knew very well this miracle would never take place — I was proven right on that point on my third, successful this time, attempt at leaving him — but this second time, in my middle forties and unemployed, I gave up once more.

At the start of the proceedings, I had told Speedy that he could have custody of the children, now teenagers, so the divorce would be less costly for him. I was so obsessed with being free of him that I was not rational. Although the children suffered from the toxic family dynamics, they had no idea the situation had a nefarious effect on me. Speedy constantly implied I was a nag, and they gratefully espoused that notion, since it gave them an excuse to ignore my endeavours at instilling in them my values of discipline, neatness, and old-fashioned etiquette, such as table manners. It made their lives easier not to listen to me. They were resentful about my wanting to leave. How could I take such a drastic step? Why would I want to leave them? I had mostly kept my mouth shut all those years in their presence. I didn't want them to live the hell I had known in my childhood, with my parents constantly arguing, my father driven to violent, frightening outbursts by my mother's passive-aggressiveness. Unlike her, I had never exploited the victim angle, and therefore they did not see me as such. On that level I was as stoic as I was in the face of physical pain. They did not perceive that their father literally drove me insane. (I would often ask myself if I was crazy.) Of course, a phlegmatic, bovine, non-analytical person would not have reacted that way to him. Perhaps, as males, our sons were bound to identify with their father. My being in school made me different from other mothers. It would take at least thirty years before the oldest two would finally understand what had driven me to leave their father. Their wives did not take to him. He reacted to one of them exactly the way he reacted to me. It would take decades and changed circumstances — cancer, family law reform, an inheritance, and steady employment — to give me the incentive and the means to successfully pursue and achieve my autonomy.

Years passed. Since 1973, I was in great pain, albeit physical this time, and I was desperate to have it dealt with. I had constant discomfort in my genital area which I could not adequately describe, over decades, to my family doctor, gynecologist, urologist, dermatologist, or internist. The latter figured I suffered from irritable bowel syndrome. His remark: "It's not what you're eating, but what's eating you." It sounded pretty astute to me. Since then, I have come to my own conclusion about the problem: it was irritable bowel syndrome putting pressure, through gas and spasms, on my bladder, which hangs down due to giving birth to huge babies, damaging the nerve endings in that area, rendering it a quivering pulp. It is a torture I live with every day, but try explaining the problem to a physician. They probably thought me a nymphomaniac because of the feeling of sensitiveness I was trying to convey.

I immersed myself in my studies and it was with great satisfaction I observed our friends' surprise when they realized I was serious about my going back to school, persisting year after year, degree after degree. They had perceived me uniquely as a sexy lady. I was showing them I was an intellectual as well as womanly. They saw a side of me they had always ignored, one of substance and determination. I dropped them as friends. I had no time for their vanities.

It made me very angry that although he knew his wife was an object of desire to other men, my husband did not bother to make himself more attentive, kinder, or to treat me in front of others as if I was someone precious. He would never walk beside me. On trips, people were always surprised to find out we were together. The only time I ever went to meet him at the airport after a three-week business trip to China — I had insisted, thinking it would be nice to make like other married couples — he barely said hello when walking into the arrivals lounge. He treated me as if I was an intruder in his world. He was still in business mode. The plane had been hours late, and I mentioned that I had been waiting a long time. That annoyed him. "You should have stayed home," he said. I was on the verge of tears. In spite of our disagreements, it could have been a pleasant reunion. I often made attempts like that at bringing some warmth into the relationship, but Speedy always pushed the buttons which turned me off. I retreated into silence. I believe he was addicted to the rush of adrenaline brought on by confrontation, his *modus operandi* with others as well, which kept me on pins and needles. On a ski trip with Club Med in St.Moritz, for dinner one night we happened to sit next to people from Germany. The moment Speedy found out their nationality he started making rude remarks referring to World War II and the Nazis. It was not that he actually hated Germans — he did business with them — but he would have just loved to start an argument. I was squirming with embarrassment. They were shocked, but did not respond and remained silent. The pre-dinner drink in our room and the wine imbibed the moment we sat down for our meal fueled his aggressive attitude. On holidays, I could never relax.

As Speedy aged, this drive for excitement through challenging others would sometimes backfire. On one occasion, as we were driving up our street not far from our house, another car coming from the opposite direction was hogging the middle of the road and did not seem to want to move over to its own side. My husband drove straight at it and was about to collide with it when the other driver realized this was a game of chicken and veered into his own lane just in time to avoid an accident. Perhaps an adoring wife would have found this a cute move. I was never relaxed enough to smile at being put in danger. "Are you crazy?" I bellowed. "Why did you just not let him pass! He looks like a biker!" I turned around and saw that indeed the other vehicle had made a U-turn and was coming back toward us. It reached our driveway, stopped, and out stepped the driver. He was burly, tattooed, ponytailed, and ranting. He did not take a swing. His parting words were "You're lucky I don't beat up on old men, otherwise I'd really give you a lesson!" Another time, as Speedy was driving up the escarpment where passing was prohibited on the winding road, he was tailed by a Porsche whose driver didn't think he was going fast enough. At a turning area in the road, Speedy let him by and then, driving right up to the Porsche's back bumper, he pushed it all the way to the top of the hill. Of course, when my husband arrived at his destination, our son's residence, the Porsche had followed him there. An altercation ensued in the otherwise quiet neighbourhood, with loud insults being directed at Speedy, again referring to his age as the reason for not killing him.

R. and his wife were mortified to the point of my son phoning and telling me about the incident created by his demented father. When Speedy was around, I was always on edge, because I never knew when his controlling *macho* pride would trigger such explosions of self-assertion and domination. I guessed this lurking feeling of fear stemmed from my father's own choleric eruptions when I was a child, which terrified me so.

A Daughter-in-Law

During that period after university and before I found employment, R., who was now in his twenties, was living with a young woman he met while on the street. She was a raving beauty, though rail thin, and a good girl. She had lodgings and took him in. K. had been born in the toughest part of town, but since the age of three until she was sixteen, she had been brought up in various foster homes because her mother had one day run away with their neighbour, abandoning her baby daughter alone in the house. The four other siblings, three girls and one boy, were in school at the time. The authorities allowed the father to keep them, but K. was judged to be too young to be left in his care without a woman around. Although later on she would see her mother occasionally, K. never forgave her for abandoning her and was smouldering with resentment. Her whole family was constantly feuding, calling each other names, "not talking," and then would be friends again. It was a phenomenon I've observed frequently with the underprivileged, as if their lives was spiced by gossip, teeming with animosity, spurred by trivialities and petty rivalries, followed by fragile reconciliations.

With this love interest in his life, R. was now grounded, and he would contact us periodically. We were introduced to K. who, with her Grade 8 education, was quite leery of us. We were deliriously happy that R. had sort of settled down. They lived together for three years in one hovel after another, and then announced they were getting married. The idea struck me as absurd. They did not have a cent, yet wanted a real wedding with all the trimmings. How to go about this was a conundrum for me. As far as life's main events were concerned, I was still steeped in tradition — French-Canadian Catholic tradition. R. was extremely self-conscious of his girlfriend being uneducated and less than articulate. Her English was of poor quality, and he would correct her every time she made a mistake. (No wonder she was ill at ease with us. I asked him to let her be.)

I gathered that if their union was not celebrated with some kind of pomp, they would take it as a reflection of the low esteem in which they were convinced we held her. Nothing was further from the truth, but I didn't see how the church wedding and reception could be achieved, since they clearly had no idea how to proceed or had the means to undertake such a project. I welcomed the adopted role of mother of the bride. I arranged for the ceremony to take place at our local church. This was no small feat, since at first the priest refused my request, given that we had not been active parishioners from the moment the children had left Catholic school. Finally, for a hefty sum, he relented. After discussing it with her, I ordered K. a bouquet, flowers, the cake, sent invitations, and took her (dragged her, really) to purchase a wedding dress. It was like pulling teeth. What could have been a joyful opportunity for the two of us to get close turned out to be a well of frustration, at least for me. K. wouldn't cooperate, dithered about letting me know her preferences, which I scrupulously sought, and did not return my calls. We had fixed a date and sent invitations, so decisions had to be made. As if they could have accomplished any of this themselves without our money. K. was openly hostile, feeling I guess like a recipient of our charity, whereas I was trying to prove to her that we fully accepted her. More than once during the various stages of the preparations I felt like dropping it all and leaving them to their own devices. Had I done so, they would never have managed to get married, unorganized and clueless as they were, insisting on a religious ceremony, not even being aware of the possibility of a civil marriage. I knew if I even just mentioned such an option, they would without a doubt have asserted that I was too ashamed of her to contemplate an elaborate, fancy event. As for Speedy, being blissfully ignorant of tradition in such matters, he was not burdened by the notion of how things should be done and did not assume any responsibility.

As things turned out, it would have been a blessing if my lack of involvement had resulted in their never getting around to tying the knot. While they were living together they quarreled, and R. would disappear for days. K. would phone our house crying, asking if we knew where she could find him. We didn't. I found those episodes very upsetting. One day she called claiming that this time R. had hit her and broken her nose. I was appalled. This was sick. As far as I was concerned, it had to stop. I felt the best, most diplomatic way to help them was to write a letter saying discord and physical abuse were not good foundations on which to build a marriage, and unless they found a way to improve their relationship, they should go their separate ways. Although I did not mention it, I wondered if two people with broken childhoods could be stable enough to build a solid life together. My intervention was ignored. The next time I saw them I searched for signs of bruises on her face but saw none. The same nose as always.

By the time the wedding day had arrived, I was convinced it was a terrible mistake, and I was almost paralyzed with anguish. After the meal in a fancy restaurant which followed the religious ceremony, the guests headed to the newlyweds' house where, according to my sisters, there was a great party. I had felt too exhausted, both physically and emotionally, to attend. We, the parents, had invited the father of the bride back to our home for drinks. He thanked us profusely for all we had done for "the kids," his financial and other contributions having been zilch. He and his daughter were practically strangers, as were her other siblings, all of whom we met for the first time on that fateful day. One of K.'s sisters, who I had been informed of shortly before, was an alcoholic and had shown up for the reception only, in gray sweats and in her cups. The first time I saw the newlyweds after their big day, K. complained the roses in her bouquet had not been fresh enough, suggesting I had stinted on the price. She said the wedding Mass was weird with the continuing standing up and kneeling down, her friends did not like champagne, and so on and so forth. When I mentioned to a colleague how my daughter-in-law never accepted anything I did for them graciously, and although I was not being generous for that purpose, a little gratitude would have been nice, he explained that she probably saw my efforts as a way of exercising control over her. I accepted his analysis. At least it was an explanation for being treated so shabbily. When Speedy, in spite of my warning him that he was wasting his time, managed to find a specialist for treating her reading disorder — something other than dyslexia — she did not show up for the appointment.

PART FOUR

A Third Career

Appointed to the Bench

That summer, after R.'s wedding, was the year I was appointed as a bilingual Justice of the Peace. I was not a lawyer, as per the British legal system, although some of us presided in court over every proceeding including bail hearings, except criminal trials and civil cases. My being the holder of a Ph.D. had guaranteed my qualifying over that of other nominees. I was sworn in and given a book of procedures to study on my own, and was told to sit in court next to the stenographer and observe the proceedings. Three times a year my fellow J.P.s and I attended training seminars. When I was introduced to my colleagues, one female, as I extended my hand to greet her, got up from her seat and walked out of the room. Ouch! Being French-Canadian, and being from the world at large as opposed to having already worked in the system in some capacity or other, where most of them were recruited, I was considered an intruder.

The other J.P.s and prosecutors — who in municipal court were not lawyers either — would get together for lunch and gossip about my performance, making fun of my mistakes once I started officiating. I know this because they never invited me to join them. Mastering the various steps and terminology of procedure was not easy. There were no rehearsals. You were learning on the job, in public. You had to think on your feet. My first bail hearing involved bestiality. My decision was not appealed by the prosecution. I had released the accused. I survived. After a few months of scorning me, my colleagues came around because I spoke English better than they did, and my humour was ruthless. They respected me, even liked me. I secretly and sincerely despised them. They were *ignorami*, philistines, rednecks, afraid of public opinion. Hence most lawyers, although groveling before J.P.s when appearing before them, did not hold them in very high esteem behind their backs. Most of them had been appointed because of their support for the party in power, such as one who was a shoemaker, or for their past experience in law enforcement, such as were ex-policemen. It made for many prosecution-oriented judicial decisions not in the spirit of the law: innocent until found guilty, which annoyed me.

I also realized that "Justice" and "the Law" are two different things. One of my colleagues, from the boondocks, with whom I shared an office — he full-time, I part-time, until he dropped dead of an aneurysm, after which I got his position — having drawn on all possible contacts, saw fit to tell me, out of the blue, that just because I had degrees did not mean I would ever know what I was doing in the job.

A stupid put-down. Knowing where it was coming from, it did not bother me unduly, but clearly I was again in hostile territory. That first bail hearing dealing with bestiality should have shown my mettle. According to what I had been taught, the accused, having no previous criminal record and being able to avail himself of a decent surety guaranteeing a reasonable sum, as well as the observance of specific conditions in exchange for his freedom, was eligible for release. With great trepidation given the revolting facts of the case, I did not remand him in custody until his trial, to the astonishment of the prosecution, who was sure that as a neophyte I would have been cowed by the scandalous nature of the case. After the events in my life, what could scare me?

My fellow justices of the peace had made an agreement with the administrative judge to throw me, although or perhaps because I was a newcomer, into bail court. My colleagues had been assigned to that court in order to relieve the Provincial judges, who until then had had to perform that duty. Bail court is very tricky and could be dangerous if a criminal is released who is a psychopath or an alcoholic with a car. Neither the judges nor the justices of the peace relished being put in that position. The presiding J.P.s preferred municipal court, located at the time in a different building where nobody noticed their very short officiating hours. I presided in bail court every day for a whole year until I realized I had been had. At that point, I claimed that I was not getting the experience in non-criminal trials which I had been appointed to hear in French. I showed my written request, addressed to the administrative judge to my colleagues so, as I stated, they wouldn't think I was doing things behind their backs. They were very impressed with my seeing through their little game. All of us then started rotating in bail court. They did not hold it against me. "Don't fuck with me" had been my message. They got it and respected me for it.

<u>Cancer</u>

During the summer of R.'s wedding, while I was in training for my judicial duties, S. was away. After his graduation from high school, I had treated him to a trip abroad as I had done for P., who traveled through Europe as intended, but S. ended up going to Asia. Before he left, I had confided in him I was so unhappy I thought I would get cancer. In September, I noticed my urine was red. I chose to ignore it. After three days it went away and I didn't give it any further thought. We were hearing very sporadically from S. and that was a worry. He was in India, Indonesia, Nepal. I knew he did not have the money for such a long period, but he was on the move, and difficult to track down. P. was already living in the United States, where he had been hired on the strength of an interview at the conclusion of his last year of university in engineering. He was doing well and had a girlfriend. It was a vast improvement on his previous life. At last, a successful development in my life!

The next April, the blood came back in my urine, but this time it was black. I was frightened. I mentioned it to Speedy, who encouraged me to make an appointment with my family doctor, who immediately referred me for an ultrasound. I was very nervous, but nevertheless I joked with the technicians who were operating the equipment. When one of them came back to advise that I could now get dressed, and that my doctor would call me, his demeanor had completely changed. There was no smile, and he was in a hurry to get out of there. I immediately suspected something was wrong. Panic engulfed me but I kept quiet. The technician having disappeared, there was nothing for me to do but wait. A week later I received a call from a woman who was the replacement for my doctor, who had gone on vacation.

She requested that I come to her office the next day accompanied by my husband. I knew right away. I asked her if the test showed a mass. "I'll not discuss it over the phone without your husband present." My husband was out of town. I insisted that she tell me the truth. She did: there was indeed what looked like a tumor on my right kidney. I made an appointment to see her as soon as Speedy returned. I got in touch with him and he took the next plane back. Fortunately, he was not overseas. In her office I explained that I had first noticed the blood in my urine eight months earlier. I should be operated as soon as possible. She was not the specialist, but she understood the urgency of the situation and my distress. Her husband, who was also a physician, happened to have his office next to that of the best oncologist in town. He would talk to him. The oncologist agreed to see me in the emergency department. "Bring your X-rays," he told me. This was done. After looking at them, he advised me to remain on the stretcher in the hall until a room became available that day, thus I would be able to remain in the hospital until surgery, which was scheduled for the next Monday. Various tests had to be performed to establish whether the cancer had spread. We had been able to procure a private room, a must for me because of my insomnia. I had a beautiful view of the blooming lilacs and hedges, the tender green of the new leaves. I would look at the people walking on the street or the hospital grounds below and think, *They and I, we don't belong to the same species anymore. Death is at my door. They're going about their routine, oblivious to their mortality.* When I had visitors (Speedy, R. and his wife, and P, who flew in from the States. After a few solicitous questions, except from my daughter-in-law, who showed no concern, they would fall back into conversation between themselves, about themselves and life in general, and I would realize how one who does not experience it cannot really perceive the reality of another's misfortune). If you've never been through it, you can't really feel it. Individuals have no imagination for or incentive to put themselves in other people's places. Hence the pro-life stance, the indifference to the plight of the homeless, to single seniors who are ill and housebound. Fortunately, the doctor was understanding enough to give me tranquilizers so the fear wouldn't keep me awake at night and depressed in the daytime. I was still aware of the noises in the hall and the regular checks of the night nurse, shining her flashlight in my face, but in a grateful state of numbness.

It was now Wednesday. Speedy contacted my sisters and Z., my friend in town. She started arguing with him about the fact that my relatives would not be coming to visit and show their support. My husband and this friend had always hated each other. They were both bullies, control freaks, and possessive. My sisters were employed, and wouldn't have spent the money on the trip. Speedy told Z. it was none of her business. They were both right: it would have been comforting to have my family show they cared at such a momentous period in my life, but it was not Speedy's fault that they didn't. Neither of us expected them to, but I didn't need to have my nose rubbed in it. Before the surgery the next Monday, I got a weekend pass to go home. Dressed in civilian clothes, I took a moment to look at myself in the entrance hall's long mirror. *You can't be having cancer*, I told the reflected image. I looked good, healthy. There was no physical pain. I didn't feel ill. The suffering was inside. As usual, though, I wasn't convulsed in hysterics attracting attention to my plight, making a spectacle of myself. I was carrying on as usual.

Upon my return to the hospital on Sunday evening, the anesthetist came in for a chat. I advised him that I dreaded being put to sleep infinitely more than the operation itself. He was very kind. The surgery took place as scheduled the next morning. There was the switch from the stretcher to the operating table, then bright lights in my face, tiled walls, masked faces leaning over me, and then the buzz of the drugs in my head reaching its terrifying climax. Oblivion. When I came to in post-op, I had the feeling I was at the bottom of a well. A nurse told me everything had gone very well, and that the doctor would be here soon. My throat felt raw and hurt like hell. I couldn't understand why. I asked why I was so thirsty. I requested water, and was given liquid but no explanation for the pain in my larynx. I found out twenty years later, when a famous person died undergoing cosmetic surgery on various parts of her body: the operation had lasted too long, and the tube providing air to her lungs had damaged her larynx to the point where she became unable to breathe.

When the oncologist arrived, he was surprised upon checking the bag connected to my bladder how active my remaining kidney was. He assured me the operation had been a success. Released from recovery, to my great chagrin and surprise, I was not brought back to my private room. In spite of my protests, stonily ignored by the orderlies, I was taken to a semi-private one. My things were already there, except for my paperback, bought specifically for my stay in hospital, which was missing. I mentioned it to my new nurse, who assured me with a straight face there had been no book. Stolen. The other bed was occupied by a South American woman who addressed me as "Ju." I had taken Spanish lessons on many occasions, but I had never heard a *y* pronounced as an English *j* before. The woman was extremely restless. She wore stiletto heels that click-clacked relentlessly on the terrazzo floor as she paced back and forth in the room. All night. She never lay down in her bed. It kept me awake in spite of my being exhausted and shot with Dilaudid.

The pain was pretty bad, cut as I had been from my navel to the middle of my back. It felt as if I had been neatly sawed in half and stitched back together again. At that time I understood that they had had to remove some ribs in order to take out the tumor, which was the size of a grapefruit. Recently my family doctor, when I complained of the pain inflicted on my torso by wearing a bra and waistband, stated that ribs are not removed in such operations, just spread apart. Perhaps he's not aware of what the technique was in 1985. Whatever. That side of my body has never been the same since. My insides around that area show metal staples when X-rayed. After twelve hours, as a matter of policy, they cut me off the opiates and put me on codeine pills, which have the same effect on me as taking cocaine. I was very agitated, and with assistance being slow to arrive, I was up the second day after the operation, cranking the handle at the foot of my hospital bed in order to adjust it to my liking, and using the washroom. The nurse couldn't get over my getting out of bed on my own. Neither of us realized my superhuman energy came from the medication.

Since the shock of the operation, the pain killers and my forced immobility had made me more or less paralyzed in the nether regions, I felt a little exercise would help my bowels. Unfortunately, as with my other surgical experiences, nothing moved. I became, as they say in the medical jargon, "impacted," an unbearable and terrifying condition which can only be resolved by manual extraction on the part of nurses wearing gloves. It has to be the most humiliating "treatment" a patient is subjected to, not to mention the excruciating pain. But what a relief after it's over. You then become obsessed with not relapsing. My family doctor, back from holiday, dropped by and informed me that he had assisted at the surgery. He mentioned that I swore in my drugged sleep and mumbled a lot. I asked what I had said exactly. He demurred with a smile, but I have the feeling I must have revealed some secrets under anesthesia.

The third day after the operation, the oncologist informed me I would be released the next day. I protested. I didn't feel ready to go home. How would I cope on my own? I couldn't keep my husband from going to work, although I knew deep down there was no point in anyone just sitting there watching me while I healed. There was no one. Two sisters had phoned after the surgery to inquire about how things were going. "Fine, just waiting now for the results of further tests, after my tumor is sliced and the pieces examined to find out what kind of cancer we're dealing with. I'm informed I'm lucky. I had a 'good cancer', so no chemo or radiation therapy is needed. Thanks for calling,"

I told them. The other sibling never called. I had tickets for a famous show in the big city within the next few days. I phoned a good friend who lived in a suburb not far away. I asked if she would like to have them, since having just been operated for cancer, I could not attend. She declined. I explained I was giving them away. She was not interested. There was no reaction at all to the cancer news. No offer to come and visit. I would have done it for her. She only lived ten miles away. I was nonplussed, hurt. She was going through a divorce at the time. The proceedings had been dragging on for years because she could not conceive being unmarried, without a man. She has complained of aches and pains forever, which are relieved only during the first month of a new romantic relationship. The laments resume as soon as the novelty wears off. She had once confided in me, as women are wont to do, that she had never had an orgasm. To this day I believe she is still looking for that moment, which she will never achieve, since her current boyfriend is in his eighties and is not "capable of much," as she put it.

The pills laced with codeine I was prescribed after my cancer surgery may have lightened the pain, but they exasperated my anger, kept me awake, with my eyes wide open all night. I was unable to relax, vociferating to myself when I was alone. After pondering my behaviour, I realized the medication was the cause of my raging state of mind. I stopped taking the pills and put up with the pain. In July, two months after the operation, I went back to my training in the courts. I had not told anyone there about the cancer, offering as an explanation a severe kidney infection which necessitated removal of that organ. This was accepted without comment. The court stenographer I had initially sat next to — actually, protocol dictated that I sit next to the presiding magistrate, but my hostile colleagues had considered this procedure of sharing the bench a bother and had relegated me to a lower tier — had been replaced by another one, new to me, but known of the rest of the staff. She was not welcoming. I noticed her hair was very sparse, extremely fine, like long fuzz. I also observed that a pile of that hair would form on the floor between our two chairs every day. Having never seen anything like it, I mentioned it to my co-workers, who laconically informed me that she was suffering from cancer and had been away for several months for treatment. She was on her third round. I could tell they did not suspect I had recently undergone surgery for the same disease. I was relieved, but that revelation, and the poor woman's condition, certainly had a devastating effect on me. She died a year later, after undergoing two other rounds of treatment, four months apart, which did her absolutely no good. She came to work until two days before her demise. She had an unhappy marriage and couldn't stand to stay home alone. Just looking at her we knew the end was near. It was a dreadful feeling, but no one dared say anything to the poor soul. Perhaps she would have welcomed words of sympathy, but what to say? It was the saddest thing in the world, the very solitary agony of another human being.

Seeing the World

Haunting me was the question of whether my own cancer would come back. It occurred to me that I should visit Africa, see it in case I died within a couple of years. I signed up for an organized tour of two countries, Egypt and Kenya. It turned out to be a photo safari. People were walking around everywhere with cameras hiding their faces, as if screwed on. I hadn't even thought of bringing one, to my fellow travelers' derision. Before leaving, I had read Norman Mailer's *Pharaoh's Evenings*, which put me in the mood for tombs and doubled my pleasure. We visited the Pyramids. Halfway up, I gave up on my attempt to climb the narrow, slanted stairs inside Cheops, my insomnia and surgery-induced weakened state robbing me of energy and making me short of breath. As we were walking back to our bus, we found ourselves beside the Sphinx. I was all set to stop and contemplate this famously ancient monument, but the rest of the group didn't seem to notice it. They were not interested. I was dumbfounded. Was it not the purpose of our trip? I remonstrated them: this was a treasure of antiquity. They wanted to get on the bus, it was not their thing, they preferred shopping.

From Cairo, where chaotic traffic made getting through the city practically impossible, lights blithely ignored by all drivers, we flew to Luxor. Our tour escort was a fortyish woman who fantasized all men fancied her and lorded it over us on that account. Lo and behold, our local guide in Luxor, a tall, thin Arab, handsome in his djeballah, with piercing and cruel, dark eyes, took a shine to me. When he brought us the gold-engraved hieroglyphic cartouches we had ordered from him, he told me in front of the others he would hand me mine in private. He took me to a café, where we had some mint tea, and asked if I would have dinner with him at his home. His family did not live there. I demurred. He understood my reluctance. No strings, he persisted, just pleasant conversation. I declined, assuring him how flattered I was, and I was. But it was risky to do so, in the sense that I did not want to get into a wrestling match. These people probably never heard of sexual harassment, the "no means no" thing. I was very pleased, however, to be able to show our delusional travel escort that a fifty-three-year-old woman was sexier than she was. I was late for our communal dinner, which was noticed by the others and reminded them I had been singled out by our local guide. Our escort was miffed. At one point, she just had to ask what was going on between the Arab guide and me. "Wouldn't you like to know?" was my enigmatic response, which left her convinced something exciting had happened. "How immoral!" was the meaning of the holier-than-thou, green-with-envy look she shot me.

In Kenya, I refrained from making a scene when our African guide "accidentally" brushed against my breast as he was helping me out of the van. I can offer no explanation why men got turned on. I certainly hadn't given any signals, not quite recovered from my recent surgery, and thought this particular male ugly as sin. I learned a few Swahili words, which one woman in our group kept referring to as "gibberish." Since I didn't have a camera obscuring my view, and being naturally very observant, I was able to spot all kinds of animals the others didn't see and I pointed them out to them. A hyena comes to mind. They marveled at my alertness. Hearing the lions roar at dawn as they were gathering at the river to drink was an awesome experience. I still relive as well the fear that engulfed me at the flimsiness of our van when we came up to the elephants in the brush and the hippos in the river. It was an experience unforgettable in its authenticity. The trip tired me, though. I took it too soon after the trauma of major surgery, but I don't regret it.

During my university years, I used some of my graduate student's grants to travel. I visited Mexico twice, Costa Rica, and Greece. I loved the sound of the ocean. My husband was not interested in sunny climes because of his extremely light complexion, which just simply burnt to a crisp. He traveled internationally to his heart's content because of his work, and did not dare oppose my setting out alone. Because of my insomnia, I never shared a room on organized tours, so I did not have a "companion." This was promptly noticed by the locals. On my first trip to Mexico, where I was visiting my mother, we went to a resort and another guest there, Hispanic, who fancied himself a poet, would come over and engage in conversation while I was sunning myself. He was encouraged to my astonishment by Mother (I think she wanted to show my aunt, who was also visiting, that her daughter was attractive). This situation also gave Mother the opportunity to converse in Spanish with this Mexican, but I was not the least bit interested. My mother could not understand why I did not respond to his advances, and I could not understand what she saw in him. He gave me a printed copy of his work.

On a trip to Greece, I had been sunning myself on some rocks, watching a bunch of young men diving into the Mediterranean. One of them came over, asked where I was from, and told me he would like to make love to me. Very much aware of the gigolo services young denizens of touristy, underprivileged countries are willing to provide to needy female visitors, I replied, in a nice way, that I was married, that my husband was a very good lover, and that I myself knew all he was after was money. How old was he anyway? This did not deter him in the least. He did not want money from me, he just wanted to make love to me. He said he would do things to me no one had ever done. He wanted so to please me. His pleas did not work. I was always terrified of catching a disease if I went with people I did not know, but it's always flattering to be desired. I asked him all kinds of questions about his life instead, then picked up my stuff and left. I never went back to the rocks. I had to satisfy myself with the pool on top of the hotel, whose water I was sure came directly from the same polluted waters as the sea.

I had befriended a couple from New Zealand, probably on the strength that being "colonials" we were different from our fellow travelers, who hailed from England, this being a British tour. This couple and I would meet before dinner, drink ouzo, and eat olives. They were almost twenty years older than me, on the verge of retirement. The husband was very attentive toward me, and, miracle, his wife showed no jealousy. We greatly enjoyed each other's company, and I felt very happy with them. One day toward the end of the trip, there was a knock on my bedroom door in the middle of the afternoon. It was the husband, looking moony. He said his wife had a cold and had sent him to ask if I had any drops. I responded "Sorry, I didn't," and did not invite him in. Looking dejected, he left, and I did not see them again until we each took a different bus after landing in London. I waved at them, and they waved back. The following Christmas I sent them a card addressed to his company in the small town on the North Island, with the word "retired" underlined after their name on the envelope. They replied, stating how surprised and delighted they had been to hear from me, and were very amused at actually receiving the card with such a vague address. Enclosed was a picture of the three of us having a drink, where we're all smiling, obviously enjoying ourselves.

I also traveled to Costa Rica when it was just opening to tourists. I had a memorable trip on a little train through the mountains which divide that small country, eating divinely sweet fresh pineapple and drinking rum. Vividly multi-hued birds and flowers came into sight as we chugged by. We also sailed to an island for a picnic, during which the young local guide who decided to keep me company claimed he was a descendant of Inca princes. He actually looked it. He was very handsome, but I was not receptive. He was offended. Later, I was sort of sorry I hadn't played the game. You can take the generation out of the girl (I don't look my age), but you can't take the girl out of her generation.

Being a Granny

After three years of marriage, R. and his wife had a little girl. I was delirious with joy since I had only had boys. My daughter-in-law's sister (the alcoholic) phoned and told me they were having a baby shower and it would take place at my house. I was not familiar with such events — I vaguely knew about them — but I never had had one, or attended one, and I was offended by her impudence. Being a feminist and an intellectual, I was against showers, bridal and otherwise. They were a manifestation of consumerism, somehow vulgar. I'd be more tolerant today. I couldn't refuse. It would have gotten back to my daughter-in-law, who would have taken it as a sign of rejection. Still, I wanted my own gift to have special meaning. I found the little silver drinking cup which had been given to the child's father when he was born, with his initial engraved on it, and proudly produced it. Its handle was broken off, but it still looked whole. The silence that greeted my gesture readily conveyed the message that they thought I was the cheapest. This was a rough bunch. They didn't like my coffee either. Two different worlds colliding. It did not occur to me then that K. would take this as an indication that I did not think she was worth spending money on her baby. I later realized that whatever attempt on my part to get closer would fail. She would always find an excuse for me not to drop in. I was dying to see my granddaughter. Whenever I phoned for news, she twisted what I said to her and I would get calls from my irate son late at night — I imagine after a scene on her part — claiming that I had insulted his wife. The one time they deigned to accept an invitation for dinner was when P. was visiting. Having served R.'s wife a well-done piece of roast beef, convinced as I was that she wouldn't enjoy a bloody morsel cooked rare the way we liked it, my gesture provoked a scene from her husband, who contended I didn't think his wife was sophisticated enough to eat her meat rare and therefore was humiliating her in front of the others. I was stunned and dismayed. I had meant well, having attempted to make sure she would enjoy the food.

At the time the little one started crawling, in order to make it more sanitary for her, I had their ancient kitchen linoleum, worn and split, replaced, at my own expense, by a new one made of smooth imitation wood tiles, which I thought would look quite handsome and go with any décor. Once it was installed, I had to phone to find out if it was done and if they liked it. The response was not enthusiastic, and we were not invited to come over and have a look at it. We were always the ones to contact them. I had also given them the furniture from my apartment in the city, which looked nice in their flat. We only saw them whenever we invited them for dinner. I missed my granddaughter; the child and I got along famously. I didn't realize until the second child was born that the bond between her baby and I rattled my daughter-in-law. About a year after the new kitchen floor had been laid down, K. mentioned that it must have been very cheap material because the corners of the tiles were now lifting. I did not see how this was possible. I had paid for quality. I accepted her comments with sad disbelief.

Having offered a loan without interest for a down payment for the purchase of a small bungalow when K. became pregnant again, we were allowed in their place sometime later to discuss the transaction. I took a look at the kitchen floor. It was as impeccable as the day it had been installed, the tiles flawless. I didn't say anything; as far as I was concerned, the situation was beyond rational. They moved to their new house, and we gave them our stove and fridge. After one visit to see their new home, we were never invited again.

My daughter-in-law chose the day we moved to the last house we were going to occupy to bring the little one in her stroller, with a little housewarming gift. It was extremely bad timing. It was four in the afternoon. I had just returned from work. The movers were still there, waiting for my directions as to where to set down the furniture. I had deliberately not taken the day off to supervise the event, not wanting to be caught in the disaster I had anticipated. Speedy had waited to the last minute to hire the movers, after I turned over that chore to him, because he had berated my choice of the ones I had reserved months in advance, claiming, among other things, my choice would be too expensive. His movers had shown up with something a little bigger than a cube van with men they had obviously hired from the street. It took them several trips to transfer our considerable household. At noon, the people who had bought our house arrived with their own stuff. Ours was not half gone. They were furious, especially when they saw one of our movers had left a gash in one of the living room walls from dropping a heavy piece of furniture.

Being tired from my day's work, upset at learning how the moving had proceeded from S., who had been helping that inexperienced bunch, angry at Speedy for the chaos that could have been avoided had he not criticized me for organizing the event, I was not at my most welcoming when K. showed up.

My daughter-in-law did not forgive me what she claimed was a rebuke of her attempt at being conciliatory. I had thanked her for the nice gesture, which in my mind had been motivated more by the urge to have a look at our new residence than by familial devotion. After all, she wouldn't allow my son to visit me on Mother's Day. The friction between us increased until a couple of years after the birth of our grandson, when she accused me of favoring her daughter and not paying attention to the boy. I explained that N. had been the first grandchild and a girl, a new experience for me since I only had had boys. I did not love one more than the other. She persisted in her accusations: I was more partial to the one than to the other. It was unfair and insane. I lost it and expressed the opinion that she was emotionally disturbed, all the frustration and resentment at my failed attempts to get close to them exploding. Accusations started flying back and forth. They walked out, the children crying, frightened. There must have been a terrible scene at their house, which upset our grandson to the point where he peed on the clothes in his drawers. This nefarious effect of our discord on the children prompted me to resolve that from now on I would just roll with the punches. I didn't see them again until S.'s wedding four years later.

R. had come over to our house a few weeks after the incident, saying he realized how our having to walk on eggs every time we were together must have been difficult, but he remained convinced I looked down on his wife for her lack of education, not just her background. I swore to him that was all in their heads, if she'd only accept me just as I was accepting her. I wrote K. a letter reminding her of the efforts, the gestures of affection and conciliation on my part, which should have proven to her I wanted a normal family relationship, that I had wished to be the mother she never had. Big mistake. The bit about "her mother" enraged her. How dare I suggest I could ever replace her mother? Her reaction was unfathomable to me at the time. Ceaselessly mulling over where it had all gone wrong, I later understood: her mother had abandoned her. What she yearned for was her real mother, not a substitute. That letter festered in her mind for years.

R. told his father and brothers I had insulted his wife. No doubt another frightful scene had ensued in their home. They believed him. It was all my fault. Speedy especially was very happy to blame me for the break up. I kept saying I understand where she's coming from, I don't hold it against her, but she is profoundly disturbed. Think of what she went through in her youth, the foster homes, maybe rape (she had hinted as much, and I had tried to learn more but R. wouldn't let her talk about it). I pointed out that R. was not a good husband. He smoked pot and drank beer all weekend, every weekend, slumped in his chair in front of the television, as she has reproached us so many times.

Addiction

It was six months after my cancer surgery when S. finally came back from Asia. His hair was shorn like a monk's, not yet the style. I mentioned my surgery, and he simply responded, "I remember you said before I left you would get cancer." S. exhibited the demeanor of a zombie. I worried to Speedy that our son appeared to be on hard drugs. I observed what I could see of his body (arms, legs, feet); no sign of needle marks. After a while, he more or less came back to normal, and left to attend McGill University. Once, when he came for a visit, I went to bed while he was watching evening television. I woke at 2 a.m., and it was still on. I came out of my room to ask him to turn it off and to get some sleep. His speech was quite slurred and totally incoherent. I was shocked and frightened. I had not seen him drinking while he was with us. I refrained from mentioning it the next day, since he seemed to have recovered, although he always sounded very confused whenever I spoke to him on the phone in Montreal.

He graduated from McGill with a degree in communications and decided to remain in that city, where he lived downtown with his maternal grandmother without any visible income. He survived on odd jobs: housepainter, mover, gofer at the National Film Board. We couldn't understand why he couldn't get steady employment. He was such a sweetie. He even took my mother for an outing from her confinement in hospital. His instability lasted until he was thirty. I had no idea what was going on. I was worried about his future, until suddenly he announced he was going back to university for a Master's in library science. His brother explained that S. had joined AA. That is how I found out he had been an alcoholic and addicted to narcotics during all those years, since his travels in Asia. They had kept it hidden from me, to spare me. I never mentioned it to S., so happy was I at his rehabilitation. I figured he had suffered enough. My equanimity surprised the boys. They expected hysterics and recrimination. They started seeing me in a different light. S. completed his Master's with great success and was immediately hired at McGill, to my relief and awe. I had taken a look at the books he had to study toward his degree. Boring and dry subject matter like you wouldn't believe. I didn't think he would persevere, but he did. I knew then he was determined to clean up his life. He soon met his future wife. She was also a member of AA, I was I told recently. She had been addicted to prescription drugs. Neither of them will touch alcohol, not even wine, even though she is European.

Tenure and Money

After much political manoeuvering, and Speedy calling on his contacts with the big shots in his company as well, I was appointed as a full-time justice of the peace. Although this support on his part was motivated by his desire to show he could successfully pull strings, an indication of his high status in the firm, a way of managing the course of my fate, I would not have achieved my tenure without his help. I was and still am very grateful to him. I had never worked for the party in power. My argument for claiming the position was that in appointing me, they were killing two birds with one stone: they were getting the replacement magistrate they needed and one who could also hear the occasional trial in French. My leverage verging on blackmail was that I could create a stink with the French-speaking community if I was passed over after four years of competently officiating bilingually. It worked. The administrative judge, who apparently did not expect me to win the competition, expressed some surprise at the effectiveness of my contacts. He had had a couple of complaints about me. One was from a cop who thought I had insinuated he was lying when he took the oath on something or other (he thought right, but I vigorously denied such a thing), and the J.P. supervisor, who felt I had not shown enough sympathy when she had endured a pre-cancer cervical test. She had led the senior judge to believe she actually had the often-fatal disease. Since he was the kind to agree with the last individual he had interacted with, he had been crestfallen by her news and appalled at my alleged callousness. He rallied after I had a talk with him and explained the nature of my colleague's medical problem. This judge was quite senile, the butt of the legal community's jokes. At the time I couldn't understand how someone so befuddled could be allowed to make decisions affecting other people's lives, but eventually I understood that by now he was doing it by rote, having dealt with the same type of cases over and over again for years. Same lawyers, same criminals. This was not civil or superior court, where they dealt with civil suits or murder. As long as the wheels of justice kept turning and the roster was covered every day, nobody complained.

That was also the year my mother died after fighting her cancer for seven years. I made the trip to visit her one week before her demise when told the end was near. I had no feelings left for her. She could have been a stranger. I went back for the funeral, not at all happy with the way my first sister, the executrix, was running things, having lent some of the inheritance money to our youngest sibling without letting the second sister and myself know. This debt had to be repaid to the estate before the distribution of the inheritance could be effected. I forgave my sister the share owed to me. It was a couple of thousand dollars. The other two didn't. I had been generous to needy people throughout my life. Except for the odd beggar on the street, I have never been shown any gratitude in return, such as asking what they could do for me. There is a cursory thanks, and my gesture is promptly forgotten. People, out of envy, resent you for being in a position of bestowing charity on them. It makes them feel inferior, but they'll take it. Some even think it is owed to them for their not being so fortunate as you. All the people on welfare I have known hated and tried to fool their social worker.

After the inheritance was divided between the five girls — our half-sister was still alive — I started decorating our beautiful new home to my taste with a vengeance: Indian rugs, the best furniture. I had waited so long to create my own nest. With my salary, as meager as it was, and my inheritance, I now had the means. Nobody could stop me. Speedy, who was indifferent to that sort of thing, was furious that I had not given him some of the money. Not a chance! For thirty-five years I had been deprived the pleasure of fixing up my home to my liking. He was making $120,000 a year to my $38,000. I went all out. People who came into the house always asked who my interior designer was. It had not occurred to them that I could have that sort of talent. Many female guests were equally annoyed that I was also a good cook. Being a magistrate, and holder of a Ph.D., it was reasoned I should be a dud on the homemaking front. Those we invited for dinner never reciprocated. After a while I realized they felt they couldn't compete. How silly of them. I didn't expect they could.

I also bought myself a gorgeous mink coat. All along I had been wearing winter ones, in which I froze and which looked cheap, because the stylish well-cut cloth ones were very expensive. I walked in the store looked carefully at all the merchandise, and found one more sporty than dressy-looking. I asked the price of the saleslady, who answered, "But that's one of our most expensive ones!" Since I didn't look like your usual rich bitch in my modest garments, she didn't think I could afford a fancy fur. "I can write you a cheque for the amount," was my response. "Immediately." Obsequiousness from the whole staff in the store ensued. They were magnificent, mahogany female pelts. Twenty-two years later, I still wear it with pride.

One of the female prosecutors in traffic court had been strutting around in a mink, with cheap coarse top hairs, lording it over me. She resented my bilingual fluency, which was better than hers. Strutting in her mink was her way of putting me down. After I showed up in my own fur coat, she never wore hers to work again. One day, I sidled up to her on the sidewalk and cattily queried, "You don't wear your mink anymore?" The look she gave me told me she understood fully my words had not been innocent. Never did she scoff again when I used refined vocabulary in court.

My friend Z., the obese one, was not happy to see my fortune change either. When she saw the mink for the first time, she inquired, "Is it rabbit?" Over the years I had put up with many of her envious taunts until one day when she was visiting — the sight of my now tastefully appointed home annoyed her — as she was about to sit in one of my living room chairs, I asked her to use the couch instead. It was more suited to her weight. She took great umbrage. I explained it was a chair from my mother, fragile because of its age, and I didn't want it to collapse under her. She could be injured. My explanation was not meant to placate her. I was making a point. In a huff, she announced she was leaving, and that I was a "cruel" creature. My exasperation with her size, fuelled by her catty remark about my mink, had been aroused by her refusal upon her arrival at my house of the diet drink I had proffered. Churlishly, she had stated she only drank pop with real sugar in it. *You're addicted*, I thought, remembering how she always went into a trance at the sight of food, or complained in restaurants that the portions weren't big enough. I had once offered to attend Weight Watchers with her, and she had refused. This time, at my house, I said, "Fine, goodbye." I had just realized that all those years I had been the one subjected to her mean outbursts. I had always made a point of sending her Happy Holidays cards. She never acknowledged or reciprocated. What was I losing by her breaking off the friendship? I don't find comfort in making people envious. I like keeping a low profile. I've learned they'll make you pay for their own perception that you're better than they are. After that, I never called Z. again. About once a year I ran into her at the supermarket and made a point of asking how she was. When I moved away, I sent her a card to that effect.

Fraudulent Treatments

The break with R. and his family was really eating at me. My insomnia was interfering with my work, which necessitated absolute concentration. I started treatment with a psychiatrist whose assistant — very nice people, they — stated that, as a condition of my being accepted as their patient, I was expected to and would be willing to participate in every step "of the programme." That was puzzling: what programme? But as I was desperate, I agreed without asking any questions. They put me on lithium. I raised the point that I understood lithium was for bi-polar unfortunates. I was depressed, down, yes, but never felt high. That was my problem: no serenity, no elation, no exhilaration. Not to worry. My medical history showed that nothing had worked so far to cure me, so let's try lithium. I was on the medication for six months. It was nightmarish. Physically, it felt as if a tremendous weight had been set on my shoulders. Any movement required a gargantuan effort. My concentration was shot. I was flying by the seat of my pants. By the skin of my teeth. On autopilot. I was terrified I would blunder in court. How was this treatment helping me? I didn't dare put an end to the torture until the day when, as part of the "programme," I had to take a very sophisticated eye test. So far I had submitted to some scans I thought were meant to determine if there was anything physically wrong with me that interfered with my sleep. This time I asked the attending doctor to explain how my vision related to depression and insomnia. "Not at all. This is just an exper..." He interrupted himself at that point, realizing he was about to give the game away. My initial flash of suspicion was confirmed. All those tests had just been research, had had nothing to do with my specific condition.

I advised my doctor's assistant of the conclusion I had reached. She didn't even deny their trickery. I added that the lithium had done me more harm than good, and that I was severing my relationship with them and stopping the medication. I was not the type to be a guinea pig, especially without my consent. She graciously received my dismissal. If they could ever be of any help, stay in touch. They appreciated me. Who had ever seen through their mercantile strategy before, had ever talked to them that way? No one. Who knew about Big Pharma in those days? I could have sued them for putting my position in jeopardy with their inappropriate treatment, but I was too unwell to think clearly. I was just relieved to banish that particular medication from my life.

Physically and emotionally, I was nevertheless still a wreck. My jaw was also killing me. In my twenties I had started getting an itch in my ears which I would try to relieve by scratching with a bobby pin. They got infected a couple of times, and I developed a red and scaly auditory canal. X-rays for the pain in my jaw revealed that long term extreme stress had caused me to clench my teeth to the extent that the joint had been injured and that it was now wrapped in ligaments, impairing its flexibility. It was impossible for me to open my mouth wide. The pain in my jaw became excruciating, especially on weekends after we had sex. It put me in a very bad mood.

I did not comprehend that phenomenon until years later. I finally consulted an orthodontist, who diagnosed mandibular disorder, and whose treatment consisted of applying hot compresses on the jaw for a period of two hours every night and repeating the phrase "I will not clench my teeth." I had one try at that nonsense, which struck me as pure auto-suggestion, utter quackery. I suppose it was very efficient with gullible souls. The guy was expensive. His greediness was confirmed when, after I informed him of my opinion on his treatment, he, without batting an eye, suggested I had crowns replace all my teeth at the cost of $32,000. This man had a great reputation in the dental community, was respected. I made sure to mention my experience with him to every dentist I encountered afterward and they were surprised. I felt he had been unethical. There was nothing wrong with most of my teeth, and my front ones were quite presentable.

The Final Break

I was constantly rehashing in mind the debacle with R. I missed my grandchildren achingly. I had counted on my closeness to them to endure in my marriage forever. In March 1990, Speedy and I left for a four-week vacation in Thailand. Since skiing was not involved, he was not enthusiastic. I asked if going away for so long could be prejudicial to his job. He assured me his decisions were not questioned at work. He had had six weeks vacation time coming to him every year for years, as he had been with the company for such a long time. We flew to Vancouver and waited five hours for the flight to Hong Kong, where the seat next to me was occupied by a Chinese gentleman who had a raging head cold and had never heard of handkerchiefs, tissue or otherwise. I had always been repulsed by people who eructed in public. For eleven hours, I was stuck next to this creature oozing germs. The irony did not escape me. When I first met Speedy, he was a spitter. "Where is your handkerchief?" I had asked him, explaining to him that this was a very vulgar habit. Disgusting. He stopped. Forty-five years later, I had a young boyfriend who didn't know any better either, but that one never listened to me. Inevitably, in that plane I caught my fellow traveler's cold.

For some reason I expected Hong Kong to be warm at that time of year. It was 50 degrees, and rained during our whole stay there. I was miserable. I had to buy a cheap plastic rain shell. On tour buses or boats in the harbour, all the guides talked about was the cost of new buildings, their size and capacity; no history. I was not impressed with the place, not being there to buy electronic gadgets. I did purchase a Chinese-style lacquered teal blue *écritoire* with an orange and yellow chrysanthemum design for our home. It was a gesture which provoked recriminations from Speedy: "Where are you going to put it?" he asked in an irate and bullying tone all out of proportion with the crime. Our huge house was full of empty spaces. My husband just didn't like the idea of my having money to spend as I chose. My new financial independence riled him.

I was in the process of making up my mind to leave him. My decision was greatly helped by the fact that contrary to our sleeping arrangements at home, while traveling we had to share the same bedroom. He was a very loud snorer, probably due to the amount of alcohol he imbibed in the day time, and any attempt at having him turn over on his side from his back provoked a very angry reaction which woke me up completely, since I had to get up from my own bed to get him to change position. I gave up and lay there, listening to this noise which had once forced P. to go sleep in the bathtub while on a fishing trip with his father. I managed two to three hours of slumber and awoke exhausted, depressed, enraged, and full of resentment toward his insensitivity to my insomnia.

After a few days in Hong Kong — the food was delicious, but to our surprise the Chinese in businesses outside the hotel were hardly conversant in English — we flew to Bangkok. It was hot, humid, and polluted, and it was where our guide met us. We were the only ones she was assigned to. She was quite fluent in English, and classy. She was shocked when I mentioned I had heard about the sexual exploitation of children in Thailand, and she vehemently denied it. I believed her. It was just a rumour amongst the general public at the time.

The Thais were small, soft-spoken, and very courteous. They were artistic in everything they touched. They handled any type of cuisine exquisitely. One evening, having dinner in a restaurant, we were served small, round dishes with tiny red pieces of some vegetable floating in what looked like water. I was about to tell Speedy I thought they were hot peppers, and not to touch them, but he already had put one in his mouth. He exploded, spat it out, tears streaming down his face, nose running, screaming, "My mouth is burning! Waitress, waitress!" I handed him his glass of water. He ranted at her, "Bring me a piece of bread, a potato! My mouth is being seared!" She didn't have a clue. She thought he was demented. We were seated in the Asian section of the restaurant, and they had no bread or potatoes. She finally understood and ran to where they served continental food and brought back a plate of bread. Speedy, thinking he was dying, raged on. I asked him what he had thought the spicy morsels were before he ate one. He liked hot foods, and this was the place for it.

We visited the city in an open boat through the canals lined with teak houses and food markets. We noticed people eating at all times of day out of a bowl whenever hunger struck. I decided we should go for a massage. The parlour was set up in cubicles; we changed into loose garments and lay down side by side on single beds for couples, then our masseuses appeared. One was of normal size, but the other weighed about 300 pounds. I thought she was the one assigned to the heftier client. No. Perversely, with a demonic grin, the big one jumped on me, walked over my back, bent my limbs backward, and cracked my bones. It was nothing like the Swedish or Shiatsu sessions I had known back home. I was terrified and she knew it. She pretended she did not understand my cries of protest. She had a porcine nose, and I could see right inside it from my supine position. In the next bed, going through the same moves, the other girl was cooing at Speedy, but with the lightness congruent to her size. After one hour, it was over. Speedy, without looking at me, got up, dressed, tipped his masseuse and disappeared, without waiting for me. I could hardly walk.

I had to tell the receptionist when taking my leave that the gentleman who had just paid was my husband. Her look indicated her puzzlement at his acting as if we weren't together. That was usual for him, insulting for me. It was like that when he had his tonsils removed. He was very annoyed that I visited him in the hospital. He had probably been flirting outrageously with the nurses. It was hard to understand. Wouldn't it have comforted him and made him proud to have his wife show her attentiveness? No, he had to look unsentimental, tough in the eyes of others, which made him insensitive in mine. Of course, I only figured that out years later. At the time it happened, it hurt.

In Thailand, we went on an elephant ride in the hills. Unsteady from sleep deprivation, I nearly fell off when trying to get onto the swaying beast from a platform. Speedy, blind to the situation as usual where I was concerned, did not offer a helping hand. For the ride aboard the elephant, we sat in baskets devoid of a protective handrail in the front. Riding up- and downhill, one had to hang on for dear life to the side ones so as not to slip out of the seat, fall to the ground, and be trampled by the animal. The handler was oblivious to our predicament. While we were in the country, a silly tourist was trampled to death by an elephant for pulling the animal's tail.

We made the trip from Bangkok to Chang Mai in a shallow motor-propelled boat with other tourists, taking our luggage with us on the craft. It took seven hours under a blistering sun, but was worth it. We got to see how the natives lived on the banks of the river, with their elephants as beasts of burden. We visited Buddhist shrines in that northern city, viewed the Golden Triangle and the Mekong River. There was no sign of life at all in Laos. We bought jewelry which later turned out to be painted plastic instead of real turquoise stone. We ventured to the Myanmar border, where I purchased a wooden statuette sculpted by the oppressed inhabitants. As it still is today, the country was closed to foreigners.

By that time I had made up my mind to tell Speedy upon our return that I was definitely leaving him. I took a good week to recover from the return flight. I had been so tense at the thought of what I was about to do that I could hardly move my legs. Although I had tried to leave him before, this time was the hardest because I knew I had the means to make it happen. The evening I was about to make my announcement, after he came home and poured himself a stiffer drink than usual, he hit me with his news: while he was away, his position in the company had been merged with another one. In other words, his job had disappeared, and he had been made redundant. Speedy had given his all to the corporation since he was sixteen. He was now fifty-eight. My shock equaled his, but for a different reason. He didn't get along with his boss, and was very demanding of his underlings, except for the women, who found him charming.

I had had to entertain some of his employees at our home and, to my embarrassment, had been asked why we had invited them. I had advised him against it, so transparent as a political move was this socializing. People were not stupid. There obviously had been manoeuvering behind his back. Someone wanted to get rid of him. I was not surprised. My husband, though honest, made people uncomfortable. He lacked authenticity. Nonetheless, I was appalled and felt very sorry for him. Under the circumstances, I could not bring myself to spring on him my decision to end our marriage. I kept silent. He did not go back to work, except to retrieve his stuff and negotiate with his superiors the details of his settlement. They offered him a very generous "golden handshake," the amount of which he finally and grudgingly accepted. They thought it was the end of it. They did not know him. He pursued the matter with threats of revealing shady transactions perpetrated by his boss. They ignored him. I kept telling him he was wasting his time, that they had an army of lawyers. His recriminations went on for years, until the company declared bankruptcy. His bitterness and drive for revenge were inextinguishable.

In the first weeks following his forced retirement, I started surreptitiously looking for an apartment. Experience taught me that a physical separation was the only way I could achieve the decisive break. I was in turmoil. I had worked up the courage to tell him I was leaving two months ago, but under the circumstances my sensitivity prevented me from doing so. He was now home all the time, telling me how to do things, such as putting the plates in the dishwasher. I was in a state of apprehensive suspension, so anxious was I to get it over with, but I couldn't bring myself to hit him when he was already down. It became so untenable I finally went to see my family doctor and described what was happening. To my great surprise and relief, instead of advising me to stay with my husband (as every other male I had consulted had done before), he thought the situation amusing. He slapped his thighs, as if greatly pleased, saying "Double whammy!" in reference to Speedy's nasty forced retirement. He was adamant: "You must think of your own well being first and carry through with your plans. Do not wait any longer."

I immediately rented an apartment downtown and hired a mover for the essential pieces of furniture I needed in my new life. Speedy's reaction to my announcement was to drink. I had pointed out our latest trip together was a disaster, and that he could stay in the house until the separation agreement was concluded. He did not take me seriously. He asked if there was anyone else. He could not accept that our marriage was a bust, and he pledged he would change his ways, that this was just a phase I was going through. When I told him I had already found a place, he relented, but the week I had to spend in our home until moving day was the longest in my life. But, as an acutely chronic insomniac, it pleased me that for once he had trouble sleeping. He received a prescription for Prozac but abandoned the medication before the three weeks necessary for it to take effect had elapsed. When all my belongings, the ones I was taking for now — I was determined to keep the house — were in the moving van, I went to tell him I was now leaving, holding my keys on the one ring in my hand. He unexpectedly grabbed it and removed the house key. I protested, "It is still my house!"

"You want to go, you can't come back!" he replied. The movers were waiting. There was no point in arguing and having a confrontation with this stubborn child.

I was away for the period covered by the lease of my apartment, one year. Once, I drove by the house and saw a white Mercedes convertible parked in the driveway. Later, upon my asking, Speedy bragged that the car belonged to a Jewish woman from the big city whom he had met on a plane — he was now a consultant in his field — and that she was a society lady, filthy rich (actually a slumlord), acquainted with celebrities. The relationship did not last. She was too independent, "wanted to do things her way," as he put it.

That summer, it rained every weekend, which did not help my mood. When not working, I was at a complete loss in unfamiliar surroundings and routine, devoid of a support system. After all, I had been married thirty-six years. I attended a therapy group for people who had lost a mate through death or divorce, but couldn't find solace there because we did not have that one thing in common: instead of being the one who had been left either through natural causes or infidelity, I was the one who had engineered the loss. Our bereavement was different. I was truly alone. I would start crying at the drop of a hat. My two girlfriends, both from out of town, came to visit and were very worried at the state I was in. My anguish was palpable, but incomprehensible to them, since my new status was of my own making. What I could not explain was that being in emotional distress was a natural, constant condition with me and the upheaval of changing my life had magnified it to an unbearable degree. My girlfriends both had boyfriends and children they could lean on. I kept telling them I was less lonely now than in my marriage.

It was not the loss of a confrontational mate which made me distraught, but the exhaustion from the effort mustered for the courage of breaking up, the legal battle which was underway, the loss of income, and the uncertainty of the outcome (since I was dealing with a most vindictive individual whose pride and wallet were being supremely injured). I would wake in the middle of the night after finally managing to fall asleep in the grip of feelings of anxiety, featuring mostly the estrangement with my son and the inevitability of having failed my life, given my disastrous beginnings. The bad memories would swirl around in my head one after another like a film, in a loop I could not break out of. Muscle spasms would ensue, wringing my back. I would get up and take ancient tranquilizers I had hoarded over the years for desperate occasions. Through heroic efforts on my part, my work did not suffer, but I was approaching the breaking point. I went to see a psychiatrist specializing in hypnotism, but that did not work. I don't think he appreciated the depth of my despair since I was my usual stoic, articulate self. Resilience. My opinions on various subjects were what really interested him, once he found out what my work and education were. Due to my medical background, family-wise, I always felt and acted on an equal footing with the profession. I was not intimidated. Some physicians appreciated it — a well-informed patient is rare and refreshing — but others resented it tremendously.

Such was the case with the next shrink I consulted, a woman whose looks reminded me of Betty Friedan's. She asked what she could do for me, as if I had entered an insurance office. An M.D. should inquire right away what's hurting you, because they are very touchy if it sounds as if you're trying to tell them what to do. Pain, apparent or not, is, after all, their business. I described my insomnia, leg cramps, and back spasms, mentioned my recent separation and the estrangement from my son, and the problems with my daughter-in-law. She saw a pattern when I described what had disturbed me about our family's dynamics: "It's not what you do or say that bothers them, it's what you are. They feel threatened. That cannot be changed, because you cannot alter where you come from, how you look, or what you've accomplished." She knew very well what she was talking about, because that's how she reacted to me the minute I walked into her office, told her what I did for a living, and related my problems in my usual articulate way. Her analysis was the same as the one I had formulated every time I had attempted to talk to Speedy about our deteriorating relationship, to no avail. It only made him furious. How could someone who saw himself as invincible admit to feeling threatened by his spouse? His resentment had been there from the beginning. This psychiatrist had now confirmed the hopelessness of it all, since Speedy would never admit to his attitude. When I informed the woman about the lithium I had been prescribed previously, she remarked it was the worse treatment for a person in my depressive condition since I was not bipolar. I needed something to lift my spirits, not to bring me down. Upon hearing those comments, I asked if she would recommend something that would allow me to sleep at night so I could muster the energy and concentration necessary to perform my duties in the daytime. "Not on your life," she said. "Should you take medication which could affect your work, you could sue me! I'm not exposing myself to that. There is nothing I can do for you!" This was brutal, cruel, and unexpected. She looked like and was a witch. The woman was clever but a sadist. She was not going to help another female as successful as she was, and better looking.

I had a friend who was an attorney in a family law firm, whom I had met when she was a prosecutor in the crown attorney's office. I made an appointment to see her in her office to ask for advice. She was very impatient with me (she was spending time on me for which, given our relationship, she could not charge me, when she could have been with a paying client, although I insisted I wanted to pay her fee). I was dismayed by her attitude. She was not that type, usually a rather classy lady. She took out the family law manual and highlighted for me the pertinent sections, of which she had a copy made for me. "You understand I can't represent you, as it would be a conflict of interest," she told me. I knew that. I was not there to retain her, I was just seeking a little comfort and support. Instead of encouraging me, she seemed to think I was a fool. When I realized she clearly did not grasp why I wanted to end my marriage, I attempted to describe Speedy's nature by relating some of his more aggressive exploits. She didn't react. She wanted me out of there. Besides, as far as she was concerned, I was so lucky to be married. She had met my husband once when I invited her to dinner, and he had fallen all over himself in his most outrageously seductive manner, as if she was Angelina

Jolie. Other men had acted this way with me and I had been embarrassed, feeling that kind of behaviour was insulting to their wives. I left him out of my friendship with her after that. I wasn't free for her in the evenings or weekends, when she would phone me out of the blue to go out with her. She must have remembered that. She had never been married, and at age forty-five, was desperate to do so. She would date coarse policemen way beneath her station. It never worked out. She had struck me as being unbalanced when it came to her romantic life, although professionally she was one of the best, albeit very restless, jumping from one practice to another every few months.

She finally married, against all her female friends' advice, a widowed childhood friend with a son. Most women aren't satisfied until they've been wedded once. She had been frantic about getting hitched. The union lasted one year. By that time she had come back to prosecuting, although she had been made partner in the family law firm. Her husband couldn't take the hours she had to put into her work and resented the prestige of her position. She was devastated by the break up and it affected her performance in court. I had no patience with her predicament. She had shown so little empathy when I was in the same situation. She had thought I was so lucky to have a man, that I was frivolous to give it up. That was an old-fashioned and dangerous mentality. Now she had a taste of the nefarious consequences of the double standard.

Sometime later, on the strength of her being bilingual, she was appointed judge in superior court. With her range of experience, she certainly was qualified, having been both a successful defense attorney and a crown prosecutor. When I congratulated her at the ceremony of induction, she hardly acknowledged me. I'm sure she found contentment in her exalted position, having finally realized that once you command an above-average salary, you don't necessarily need a man to have a life. She had been saddled with student debts until then. At the beginning of our friendship she had mentioned how much money she owed, and I was shocked. She wore designer clothes. I had been reminded of how I had been denied a career for lack of funds and of knowing the ropes.

By inquiring of the court stenographers who rotated between all the courts and thus got to know how the various actors in the system operated, I got the name of a divorce lawyer who was supposed to be good. On our first meeting, he went through the usual routine, saying that maybe I should work things out with my husband and forget about leaving him, since he did not beat me and was opposed to the idea. This time I stood my ground, but I warned the law man that Speedy would be extremely difficult to deal with and it would be a laborious process. Mr. Lawyer did not believe me: "We have family law; your case is straightforward, no problem." I informed him that my husband had decided to represent himself. I had warned Speedy that judges, who are lawyers themselves, do not relish having to deal with people who do not hire attorneys, especially if those people are not poor, but my advice was ignored. Speedy was convinced he always knew as much or more than anyone else (which was correct, in certain fields). This information was meant to give Mr. Lawyer an idea of what type of individual we were dealing with. I assured him he had never before encountered a character like my husband. "Not to worry," was my counsel's attitude. I had asked him, in order to soften for Speedy the finality of this drastic step I was about to take and thus not provoke him any further, to work out a separation agreement first before moving on to divorce proper. Speedy was served the papers and immediately contested the terms, arguing that under our marriage contract, entered into with my father in 1954, in another province, all he owed me was $10,000. We had to go to court for him to be told by a dismissive judge that the said contract was not recognized where we now lived. This pronouncement confirmed what my lawyer had already stated in writing.

After losing that first round, Speedy retained a lawyer, having realized from the judge's attitude that he was not helping himself by appearing in court without a specialist of the law at his side. Unfortunately, he did not listen to his advocate, but rather told him what to do. After receiving the information from my side on how, according to family law, our property and assets would be divided, he had his own lawyer send us his very tortuous, convoluted diverging calculations, pages and pages rationalizing his computations, reams of paper, which my attorney dutifully read, and charged me for the time he spent doing it. The whole process which should have taken three months at the most, and cost me no more $1,000, was now into its sixth month, with fees mounting.

Initially, my lawyer had reasoned that after thirty-six years of marriage and raising three children, I should ask for alimony, my income being so small compared to Speedy's, but I had declined, in order not to complicate matters and delay the outcome, but he no longer insisted, having now had a taste of Speedy's tactics. After more haggling back and forth and getting nowhere — my husband was not about to sign — it was now ten months since my first appointment with the lawyer, my attorney decided it was time to go back to court to resolve matters once and for all. I was a basket case. My husband was claiming the settlement agreement I had entered into at the time of our second separation was valid, although that had been arrived at before the new family law had come into effect. In court, his attorney dutifully stated to the judge what Speedy's perception of how our property and assets should be divided. The magistrate's response was unequivocal: "Shame on you, Mr. Wilson, you should know better than wasting the court's time like this. This will proceed according to law." And that was that.

In exchange for Speedy letting me keep the house, I agreed to forego my share of the national pension plan, which was considerable, since he had been working since he was sixteen and had been earning a good salary for years. I, on the other hand, had only been employed full-time for two years at ridiculously low remuneration, but I was entitled to equalization, which would have deprived him of a certain income he felt was coming to him alone. I pointed out to him he should count himself lucky I was now working, otherwise he would have had to continue supporting me in the manner I had become accustomed to. But he was deaf to that logic, determined to make things as difficult for me as possible.

Ten years later, when I retired at the age of sixty-eight, in the course of an interview with a government official regarding certain forms I had to fill out, she informed me that no matter what had been stated in the separation agreement the law provided that I get the benefit of equalization regarding my estranged husband's national pension. By that time, I had gotten over the emotional turmoil of our separation and was all for this benefit in my favor. I was no longer afraid to play dirty. Speedy admitted he had been aware all along of this quirk in the law, but he was not about to let go. Back into court we went. He lost again, for the simple reason that we were now living in another province. Our separation was not even valid there without a judge's approval. If I wanted to, I could be mean and greedy and start the process all over again, to my advantage.

Before signing the definite document, Speedy had insisted on my paying him half the amount he estimated the house was worth, way above its value at the time. Thanks to my inheritance, I had the necessary funds to do that, but when the place was sold ten years later, just before the boom, it was for a price much lower than what his assessment had been. My lawyer disapproved of my being so conciliatory, but I had had enough. I wanted to get it over with, to be done with the wrangling. He relented, reflecting that Speedy was a pompous bastard who would not hesitate taking the matter to the Supreme Court if I did not compromise and allow him to save face. The lawyer acknowledged I did not have enough years left or the means to pursue the matter. I let Speedy calculate the value of our furnishings, which had all been purchased with my money. At that point I couldn't be bothered. Whatever. When the lease for my apartment was up I moved back into the house and he rented his own place in another part of town.

I immediately left on a three-week trip, a Mozart tour, that year being an anniversary of the musician's death. We visited all the cities where he had lived. I, by myself of course, basked in the relief of being free of the uncertainty and stress of the past year. I felt guilty at having left my husband, but at the same time I was elated that he was no longer by my side, spoiling my trip. I certainly would never forgive him for not bowing out gracefully and generously.

On that tour we visited countries I had never traveled through before. This was 1991; the contrast between what had been West and East Germany was still striking. At the border of Czechoslovakia, which had even more recently thrown off its communist regime, our bus was stopped. We were told to get off, and our passports were collected. It was 90 degrees outside and there was nowhere to go but a little variety store just inside the border. It carried brands of candy bars which tasted as ancient as their wrappers looked. The local red wine was seventy-five cents for a big bottle. There was no beer and no soft drinks. They ran out of the only food, sausages. The day grew long and sweaty in the blazing sun. Some of my fellow travelers started complaining loudly. I told them to shut up if they did not want to be detained indefinitely by these very officious, self-important, and no doubt envious of our Western freedom and affluence civil servants, who could also decide to refuse us entry if we displeased them. I could sense democracy had not quite yet implanted itself in the minds of these border guards. We were entirely at their mercy. Finally, I was called by our tour escort, who held my passport in his hand. "Your form indicates you're a judge," he told me. "For you, there is no problem being admitted into this country. You're the first one." The rest of the group was then admitted each in turn.

On that trip, a concert featuring Mozart's music almost every evening was the norm. In Vienna, we attended an opera, *Rosenkavalier*. Those of us who traveled as couples were treated to good tickets in the orchestra and mezzanine. The single women, like me, were relegated to the top tier known as the *poulailler* (the henhouse in French), where there are only wooden benches against the back wall, and a railing over which those who have to stand can lean; otherwise, the stage is invisible, though you can hear the music. The *habitués,* having grabbed the benches, followed the melodies in a book without bothering to get a glimpse of the stage. The novelty of the experience kept my outrage at being so treated at bay — we had all paid the same price for tickets. During intermission, we went down to the bar and enjoyed the parade of elegantly long-gowned Viennese ladies who were regular patrons of the opera.

The last venue was in Paris, in a chapel which had no air conditioning. Our group of tourists was seated on one side of the center aisle, Parisians and other assorted Europeans on the other. I found it interesting that the former were desperately fanning themselves with whatever was at hand. They were very uncomfortable in the ambient heat, whereas the locals did not seem the least bit indisposed. As was I. I dislike air conditioning, being very sensitive to the cold. I took the opportunity, while the rest of the group toured famous sites in Paris — their first visit to the City of Lights — to hurry to the newly-opened Musée d'Orsay. During my previous stays in Paris, I had never deigned sail down the Seine on a river barge, a favorite of tourists, which struck me as tacky, costly entertainment, but this time it was included in the tour. It was a midnight cruise. There was a full moon, and luscious summer weather. I was struck and moved by the beauty of the illuminated buildings along the banks. What I had expected to be a clichéd attraction turned out to be a sensuous and unforgettable experience.

A Professional Nightmare

Upon the first morning of my return from that trip, as I was looking forward to enjoying my home again, shopping for furniture to replace what Speedy had taken with him, and still suffering from jet lag, I picked up the paper on my doorstep and glanced at it, intending to give it a full read after dinner when my daily obligations had been fulfilled. It was sort of a reward at the end of the day, reading being my favorite pastime. I never gave in to instant gratification, as had been instilled in me during my disciplinary upbringing. What I saw on the first page chilled me to the bone. One of my worst nightmares had come true. It was a professional nightmare this time: an accused person I had released on bail a month earlier on charges of gun possession and sexual assault had just murdered the daughter of a prominent surgeon. Cornered by the police in a car chase in a shopping centre parking lot, he turned the gun on himself, committing suicide. His death required a coroner's inquest.

His lawyer had not called his client to testify in his bail hearing, knowing full well the accused was mentally disturbed and would have been remanded had he taken the stand. The presumed victim of the sexual assault that brought him to court gave very dubious evidence, considering that the next day after the offence allegedly happened she let him into her house again, and only called the police when she noticed he was armed. The woman was to later get in trouble with the law herself. I had not thought her credible. I released the man on the promise of his lawyer that he would immediately take him to a psychiatric facility. That was done, and there he remained under observation for a month. Since he had committed himself voluntarily, they released him after that period, not perceiving him as a danger to himself or others. That is when he murdered the girl. The mother of the victim blamed me publicly for having released him on bail, as did the head prosecutor. Relentless articles in the papers claimed J.P.s were not qualified for dealing with criminals. I had the support of my colleagues and the judges who knew I had done everything by the book. Unfortunately, the public does not know the book. I maintained my composure and carried on as usual, realizing the coroner's inquest, which would take place a year later, would reopen the whole can of worms. I was shunned by the defense lawyer who, when I first ran into him after learning the terrible news and asked him what went wrong, didn't he know his client was crazy? replied curtly that he and I shouldn't be seen together, that *he* was in the clear, and had consulted those in the know, that *he* as a defense attorney, who must think of his client first, had acted legally.

The Home Stretch

That Christmas, I had Speedy, P. and S. over for dinner. At the table, my husband (after many glasses of wine) suddenly started blubbering that their mother was breaking up the marriage, that he loved me, and that he had done nothing to deserve this. Seeing him in tears like that reminded me of Father, a monster who had never cared about his children's welfare, but who could get very emotional over some historical fact or figure, and whom I felt like slapping in the face on such occasions. Where was his concern for his daughters, starving for affection? Those tears never elicited my sympathy. Our sons must have thought at that moment I had a heart of stone, but alcohol had a lot to do with bringing the self-pity to the fore. Speedy had finally realized with the signing of the separation agreement that my decision to leave him had not been a sudden, capricious impulse on my part, and that I would not "come to my senses."

The boys were not aware of the excruciating process which had taken place in the last year. In fact, they had not understood that all those years I lived with him, their father literally drove me crazy. This scene at the Christmas dinner made them feel very bad, very sorry for him. They saw me as the villain, definitely. I was a bad person, responsible as well for the estrangement with R. Later on, P. declared, on the phone, that if I got lonely in my single state not to expect any sympathy from him and not to come whining. It had been my choice. My sons were angry at me, although they were adults by now. At the time, P. did not put two and two together, not even when he decided to stop going on fishing trips with his father and S., for the reason that when Speedy had a few drinks in him, he inevitably picked fights with them. His snoring would keep them awake as well, as it had done me. It was an unpleasant togetherness they could do without.

I was very much alone. Outside work, I had nothing in common with my colleagues, who were all married anyway. My two best friends who lived out of town had boyfriends. I agreed that summer, when Speedy's lease was up, to have him live in the house until he found lodgings in Montreal, where he had decided to go back to live his retirement. He also persuaded me to go for marriage counseling in a last ditch effort to mend the marriage. I may have been lonely, but I was not as miserable now as when I was expected to have sex with someone I couldn't stand and did. I wasn't living in an atmosphere of constant confrontation. I told the therapist in front of my husband that since Speedy was the one who wanted to be married, he was the one who had to change. After thirty-six years, I had absolutely no interest in making any effort in that direction. No matter what I did, Speedy would always resent the fact that I was not stupid or submissive, that I had a Ph.D., that I had a prestigious position while he no longer had a job, and that he had no cultural knowledge or interests of his own, not to mention his excessive drinking and insane driving. I craved the seaside and the beach. His complexion did not allow him to go outside in the sun.

In the counselor's office, my husband denied and pooh-poohed all my complaints relating to his behaviour. How can one change something one does not admit? Around the third session, the therapist's first question was "How did the weekend go?"

"Very badly," I replied.

"Tell me about it."

"I asked Speedy to wash the three windows in the house, and he refused and became very angry when I insisted. I always do the four sets of French doors myself, because they're much more work and hard on the fingers since they feature small square panes of glass."

The counselor said to Speedy, "Why would you refuse to do that? It's not an unreasonable request."

His reply: "She's just a nag."

Rain was streaming out of our skylights into the house as if there was no glass, not just leaking. They needed to be looked at. I thought he should see to it, but he refused, absurdly insisting it was mere condensation. I declined further counseling. We weren't getting anywhere.

That summer, the coroner's inquest into the death of the murderer I had released from custody before he committed his crime started. The government provided me with a lawyer, their lawyer, a brilliant and extremely good looking man from the big city, who was well aware of his attributes and behaved accordingly. He was already busy with another murder trial somewhere up north, which he was not about to neglect to represent me. He sent someone else to stand for me in his place at the inquest. He would phone me at home every night to give me advice and report on what had taken place as he had heard it from his representative at the hearing. He enjoined me to not speak to journalists, arguing that if I gave in, they would never let go and exploit the situation. He didn't have to tell me that. I was well aware of the ramifications my consorting with the press could conjure. If digging into my past they had found out that my son had done jail time for vandalizing, my goose was cooked. Especially since the mother of the victim had become a publicity junky. She had founded a movement for stricter gun legislation, and was openly blaming me for the death of her daughter, supported in this by the head prosecutor, who was happy to deflect the blame away from his office. He told reporters he had looked into my record at traffic court and found it wanting.

Of course. I was known as defense-oriented: I was not an ex-police officer or court clerk who had always been paid by the system and was owned by it. Neither was I a political appointee, a civilian who had only a vague notion of what the concept of innocent until proven guilty meant. My neighbours were even making remarks in my face: "A justice of the peace is not well trained enough to judge in court." Had anybody cared to research it, they would have found that judges always released people who came before them with a dated and minimal record. After all, that is how I had learned, sitting in on bail hearings presided by judges, before they got me to do the job (which they hated, because it was not safe).

One day crossing the street at a busy intersection, I was hit in the ribs with an elbow by a criminal I had remanded in custody and who, having pleaded guilty and done brief time, was now free. He remembered me denying him his release and that was his way of exacting revenge. Fortunately, there were dozens of people around, otherwise who knows what he would have done to me. And what is case law mostly based on but mistakes committed by first instance judges? During the coroner's inquest, no one insisted on the fact that psychiatrists had let the murderer go after a month's close observation in a mental institution. That would have been my lawyer's argument, but he was not there. My superiors were proud of the fact that an expensive attorney had been provided for me, but I felt he did a lousy job by not pointing out that if the medical profession did not see that the murderer was a dangerous individual on the brink of going over the edge, how could anyone else? I did not expect the general public to understand the intricacies of the law, but I was sickened by the treachery of the head prosecutor. A few years later, when this same man had to attend in my court on a rotation basis after obligatory retirement, a catty court stenographer volunteered the opinion that if she were me, she would refuse to work with him. I replied that I didn't care anymore, but I made sure to spell out his mistakes whenever he lost his cases before me, to humiliate him to the hilt. He couldn't touch me. In criminal court, my judgments were never appealed, my arguments very tight, and my decisions always resting on solid ground. The real reason I did not make a fuss about having to work with this treacherous individual was that had I declined to preside on the days he would appear before me as prosecutor, I would probably have been relegated to work in the office doing paperwork, another J.P. would have had to be found at the last minute to sit in court in my place, jerking the inertia of the bureaucrats who set up the schedules and making me a nuisance. I might have ended up taken out of bail court altogether. I'm not one to cut off my nose to spite my face. Long-term vision, that's me. Another aspect of resilience. It was summer, so I kept my mouth shut under the persecution, but I did ask for a two-month stress leave, which was granted. My colleagues could not believe my low-keyed reaction to the calamity that had befallen me.

Speedy was acting up, resenting the daily phone calls from my lawyer, reverting to his old jealous, controlling behaviour. Since, at the time, we were still attending marriage counseling therapy together, when he went to an ISO conference in Brazil I accompanied him. It was a good opportunity to see Rio. We stayed in a hotel on the beach near the Sugar Loaf, but not the one known as Ipanema. I was warned not to venture out of the hotel on my own, that it was too dangerous. It was like being a prisoner while Speedy was at his meetings. One day around noon I decided to go out. I walked on the boulevard between the hotel and the beach as far as the Sugar Loaf, watched the sky divers, and then, on impulse, reasoning I couldn't visit Rio de Janeiro without having treaded upon the sand, I came back along the shore, absentmindedly taking in the near-naked sunbathers and the ocean, daydreaming. I had almost arrived in front of my hotel when I realized I was surrounded by a bunch of youths in their late teens. One of them casually lifted my arm, unclasped my watch, and took it. It was a cheap watch but expensive-looking. I did not fight back. I remained calm, although I wondered what they were going to do to me. I was at the center of their group, hidden from view. The young man was talking to me in a soothing tone, in his language, which I did not understand but it seemed to me he was saying he was not going to hurt me. Another one took my fanny-pack and opened it. I had been careful not to carry any money, just the case for my sunglasses. Seeing it held no valuables, they gave me back the pouch and dispersed. I looked around. The beach dwellers did not seem to have noticed anything. Pretending, most likely. Mugging tourists was common practice in Rio. I went back to my hotel somewhat shaken and asked security to advise the police of what had happened. I'm sure they thought I was an utter fool to have stepped out alone. I had heard stories of being mugged even murdered in Brazil, but you always think these things happen to someone else. I was not unduly upset, however. I choose to look upon such incidents as redistribution of wealth when visiting poor countries. We had planned to rent a car and visit the countryside, but it was now out of the question. I didn't want to get killed.

When we came back home, I asked Speedy to leave the house, stating that the marriage was definitely over. He bought a condo in an upscale neighborhood in Montreal, in the same end of town where he was brought up, except now on the better side of the tracks, and he promptly started dating the building receptionist. On the day in January he had picked to move out with his share of the furniture, I took a look at the truck and wondered if it would be big enough. If not, it would delay the final moments of what were necessarily to be very awkward and harrowing hours for both of us. They managed to get everything in except the teak dinette set, made up of four chairs and a rectangular table. I offered to buy it from him. I was fond of that furniture I had picked myself, and I knew I wouldn't be able to find the same style and quality again. Speedy rejected my offer. "But there is no room for it in your condo!" I had seen the place, and my father's big oak roll-top desk was going in the space meant for eating near the kitchen. He was adamant I was not getting the dinette set, that I would have to buy a new one. The movers had to repack the truck and finally managed to fit it in, the doors barely closing. It was typical of my husband to deny me to the last minute, to assert his will. That last petty gesture made parting easier for me in the end. Thirty-six years it had been. I was now fifty-eight. I found out later Speedy had given the set to his girlfriend's niece.

EPILOGUE

All through writing this memoir I had the feeling, nay the certitude, that I had survived enough adversity to be guaranteed sweetness and grace from age seventy-seven to my dying day. Well, as I have often stated when I hear the phrase "It can't get worse," things can always get worse. Fate has now proven me right. For the second time, I have been subjected to the worst misfortune to strike a woman: I have lost a child, suddenly and irremediably. I don't know if I have enough years left to experience closure, but at that fateful moment it appeared that his death might bring me back the son I have been estranged from for decades. That estrangement was really my first loss because it also deprived me of the presence and love of my grandchildren. I have been able to cope with those tragedies by telling myself they were just retribution for not being the attentive mother I had wished to be. "What goes around comes around" reasoned the philosopher in me to parry the distress. The sleep disorder had determined my moods and affected my behaviour, but I find consolation in the fact that none of my three sons were/are afflicted with the plague of insomnia, that two of them achieved good marriages and successful careers. Two out of three ain't bad in the circumstances. They, in turn, were/are proud of my accomplishments, as I, which brings me serenity. I will die fulfilled having run the gamut of human experience.

That would be the answer to why decrepitude has not touched me.

CPSIA information can be obtained at www.ICGtesting.com
Printed in the USA
LVOW080732300513

336031LV00002B/27/P

9 781622 128075